POULTRY GUIDE POST

BELIEVE ME!

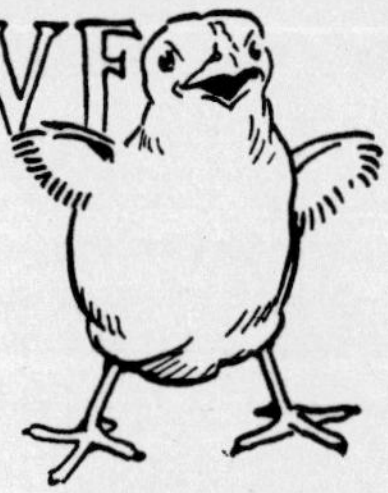

POULTRY GUIDE POST

BY

PHILIP R. PARK

ILLUSTRATED BY

HENRY C. GROVER

PUBLISHED BY
THE PARK & POLLARD COMPANY
BOSTON, MASSACHUSETTS

PRESS OF
THE KENNEBEC JOURNAL
AUGUSTA, MAINE

FOREWORD

WHILE the terms used in the following pages are in most cases descriptive of common articles of trade, the names may be new to some of our readers so we take this opportunity to explain our meaning more clearly.

Egg-Feed as used herein refers to a mixture of ground grain, corn, wheat, oats, barley or kaffir corn mixed with mill feeds, bran, middlings or shorts, ground Alfalfa, a little salt and some animal matter like meat scraps or finely ground fish, (a non oily variety preferred). This mixture is not to be fed wet but absolutely dry in proper dishes or feeding devices kept constantly before the birds.

Scratch Feed is the name used for a combination of wheat, oats, barley, cracked corn, buckwheat, kaffir corn and sunflower seeds. Other combinations may be used and the proportion and quantity of the grains will necessarily vary from time to time, with the market. Always be careful that the feed contains nothing musty, mouldy or tainted.

Chickfeed means a mixture of small sized cracked grain and seeds, and usually consists of cracked wheat, corn, kaffir, millet, canary seed, oats,—and in some of the best a little dried fish, which acts as a relish and stimulant.

Growing Feed is a mixture of whole grains ground together with meat food added before grinding. It makes a wonderfully effective feed when properly prepared.

CONTENTS

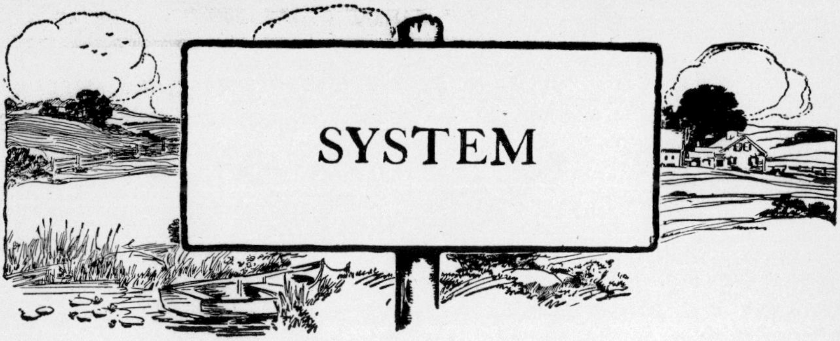

SYSTEM

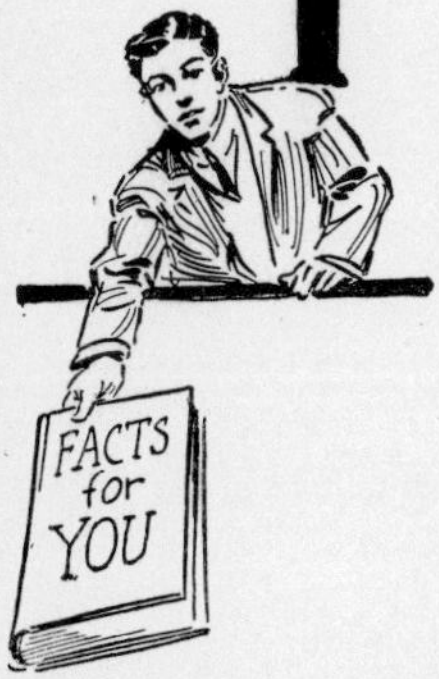

YOU have all heard of the famous sayings of Louis D. Brandeis, during the recent rate hearings before the Interstate Commerce Commission at Washington,—that he could show the railroad managers of this country wherein they could save a million dollars per day in their expense accounts.

We are equally certain that we could show the poultrymen of this country wherein they could save for themselves an equal amount, and when saved it means much more than the corresponding increase in their profit account, for in many cases it signifies the doubling or trebling of the profit, and in most instances, the turning of what had been losses into good profits.

Professor Adams, of the Rhode Island Agricultural Experimental Station, recently made the statement that if the corn growing literature and lectures going on in this country had increased the yield one kernel per ear, this added increase would amount to $1,800,000.00 in the pockets of the farmers of the United States.

Fresh Air for your Birds.

Now we are going to show you where you can increase your efficiency 10% to 50%, and if this is extended to every poultryman in the country, the added revenue would amount to more than the National House of Representatives could spend in a double session working overtime.

And why should not the poultryman take just as careful a survey of his losses and drawbacks as the business man? Think of it! Probably the average large business of this country is done on a less than 5% net profit, and it is safe to state that the dealers in feed stuffs and the necessaries of life, get less than 2% net profit.

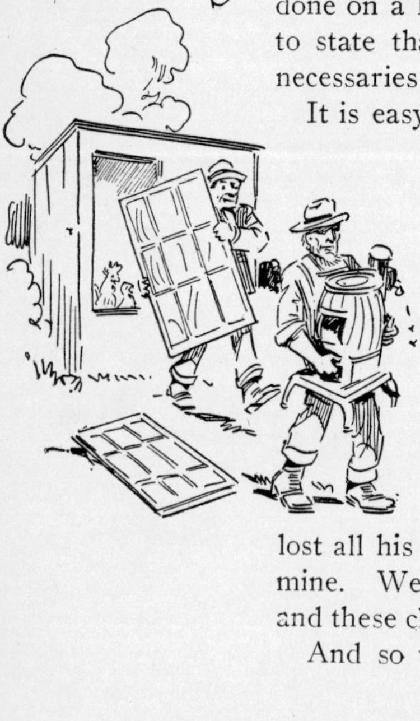

It is easy to see that these business men could not allow a loss in the process of manufacture of 90%—nearly equalling their total sales. They would be camping on the trail of the foreman who allowed any such waste of raw materials, and they would camp there just long enough to get a new man for the job. But we poultry raisers, in our optimistic manner say,—"Well, I am doing better than Bill Smith, because he lost all his chickens and I only lost two-thirds of mine. We will run the incubator another hatch and these chicks will only be three weeks behind."

And so we excuse ourselves in the most diabolical slip-shod fashion, and content ourselves with records because they are no worse than the other fellow's.

We have no knowledge of any business outside of highway robbery that could stand any such losses as the poultrymen experience year after year, and swallow with apparently little, or no thought. For instance, not many years ago the writer was called to suggest a remedy for a plant that was losing a large percentage of its chickens before they were three weeks of age. In the course of the conversation, in getting the facts of the case, the owner made the statement that he had hatched that season 15,000 chicks,—and he had raised less than 1500! Nevertheless the plant is still running. The owner is still in charge. It must be paying or there would have been a change of ownership before this time. Another owner made the statement that he has been raising chickens twenty years, and he would guarantee that he had buried as many pounds of poultry as he had marketed!

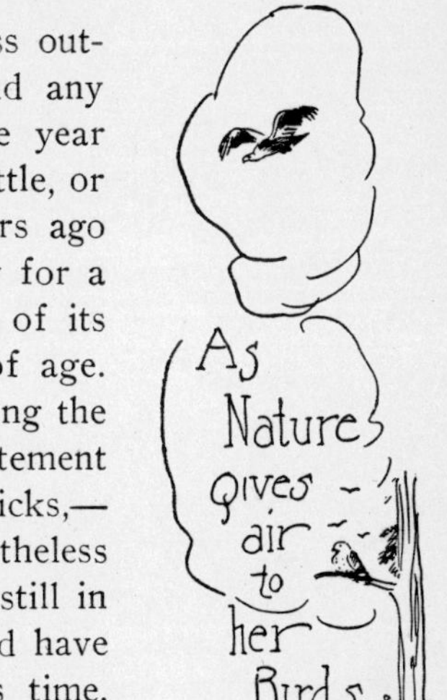

Did you ever stop and consider that there is a right good reason why every egg does not hatch, and an equally good reason why every chick that chips the shell does not grow to maturity? And the chances are that you are just as innocent as guilty of this frightful mortality.

You, in your enthusiasm, want to take particularly good care of your breeding stock, so with great pains, much time, and some cash, you very carefully cork up any opening of any kind in your poultry house. You feel that you are doing them a particular kindness, and you see to it that the wind is tempered, and that your pets never get out of doors on the cold ground in anything but pleasant weather.

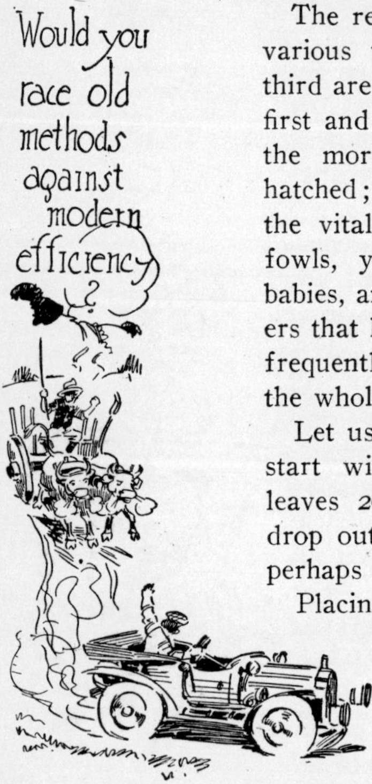

The result of this smothering is seen in your various tests of eggs in the incubator. One-third are not fertile. One-third die between the first and second tests, a 25% hatch results, and the mortality keeps right on after they are hatched; for not having yet been convinced of the vitalizing effect of the air upon your old fowls, you are equally painstaking with the babies, and they are kept in super-heated brooders that kill off all but the very strong, and quite frequently make a good clean job of it—and take the whole lot.

Let us see how this will figure out. We will start with 300 eggs. One hundred infertile, leaves 200 in the machine, and 100 of these drop out before the final test, and we get out perhaps 75 chickens.

Placing these in heated brooders that have always killed more or less, we find that we have 35 chicks of two pound weight to go to the roosting coop or market, and we will call them worth 50c. each.

Now we will start on the increased efficiency plan with an equal number of eggs, but these eggs were laid by hens kept in open front houses — same houses costing less than the other kind, — the open air treatment resulting in greatly increased vitality. We find only 10% of the eggs infertile, and we only lose about an equal number between the first and second tests. This leaves about 250 eggs in the machine, and when the hatch is due we get a full 200 chicks that are full of ginger and snap.

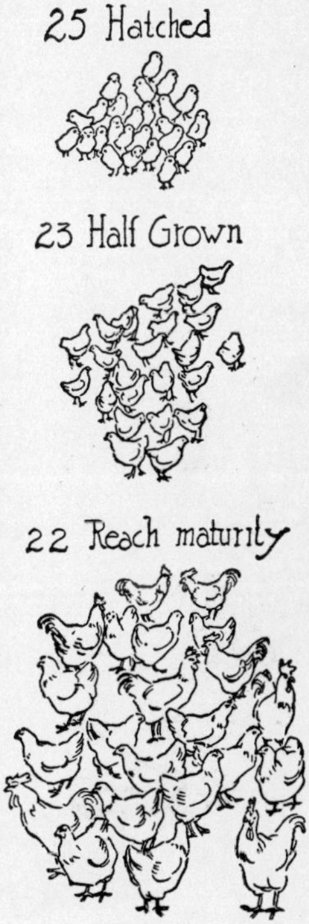

Here we find the increased efficiency program has given us 200 strong, hardy chicks from the same number of eggs, the same care and attention that yielded us only 75 second grade youngsters on the old style plan.

In brooding the babies after they are hatched, more wonderful and startling comparisons are found. We place the 200 efficiency chickens that have started life's battle with a strong determination to live, in eight heatless brooders and follow directions. Here the air conditions and heat conditions are almost identical with Nature's own methods, and at the end of three weeks we have 100 chickens, while with the 75 chickens in a heated brooder, heated to a degree recommended by the manufacturer, and maintained with greater or less success—it is usually found at the end of three weeks that we have about *half* as many chickens as we started with, and we pass it up as the usual mortality, and go on grinding out more to run the same gamut of trouble.

The modern higher efficiency method costs much less to install and has everything to recommend it so far as economy of time and expense is concerned, and you may well ask, "Why

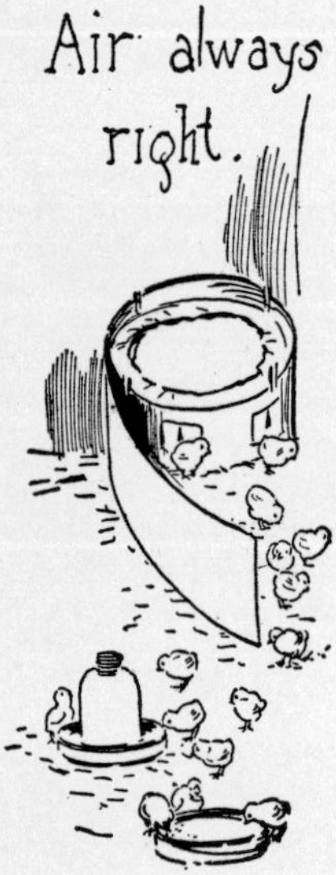

do the other conditions exist?" The only answer is, "The skeptical mind of the public."

So much for the difference between the housing of the old breeding stock, and the brooding of the chickens up to three weeks of age.

Comparing the Feeding System, we find a still larger waste that could be corrected. The average method of chicken feeding is on the plan of keeping the chickens hungry, relying upon their keen appetites to correct the inefficiency of their diet. They feed boiled eggs, cracker crumbs, corn meal, oats, johnny cakes, cracked corn, meat scraps, wet mashes, and many other combinations, alternating between half starved conditions and five-minute gorging processes, that pass as feeding time.

As against this we have the modern efficiency method, using Growing Feed, which should be a combination of meat and grains ground together into a most palatable ration, kept always before the chickens from one week's age to maturity. This feed is always within easy access of the entire flock. Each member has forty feeds or more per day, takes it as his appetite craves, and finds an unending supply. Never from the end of the first week does any member of the flock realize what the pangs of real hunger mean. The result is: market chickens in beautiful condition two weeks to two months ahead of the old plan chickens, and pullets from one to two pounds heavier at the same age, rounded out before laying as perfectly as yearling hens.

Did you ever stop and consider the various processes that the feed goes through in the digestive economy of a chicken? We think it is not recorded who first advocated feeding ground feeds wet to poultry, but we all did it, and many of us are doing it today.

Why? Because our fathers and mothers did it. Now, we all admit that the best laying and the best growth cannot be obtained by feeding hard, unground grain, because we have so developed the birds' appetites that their intestines are capable of digesting the food much faster than the gizzards can break up and grind whole grain.

Thus, we find that growing chicks, or laying hens, make much more rapid growth, lay more eggs or make a more complete development when fed ground grain. The reason, as we see it, is as follows: When fed on wet mash in the morning they gobble down a cropful in five minutes or less time; practically no saliva is mixed with the food in the process. This cropful of food is mildly attacked by the juices of the crop, which can only penetrate the outside of the mass before the inside sours. The passing of the food through the mouth so rapidly, and the gorging of the crop, practically throws all the work that should have been done previously, upon the intestines.

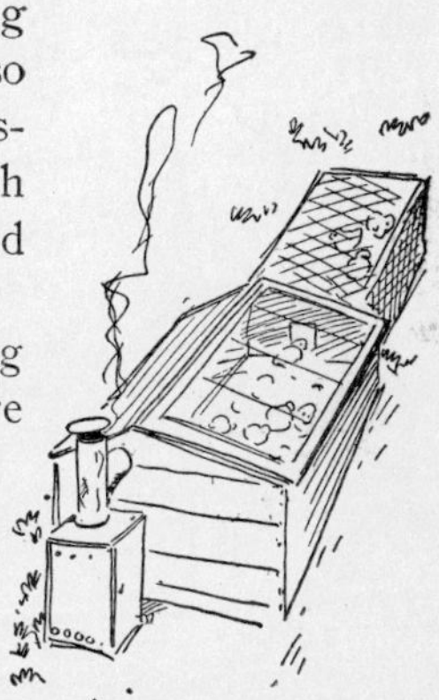

Air never right.

In this way less of the food is digested, and more or less irritation arises, causing a tendency to bowel trouble, and less efficiency in the number of eggs and growth of the bird.

Now, when the birds eat ground Growing Feed or Egg Feed, they take the feed very slowly, mixing it thoroughly with the saliva before swallowing, (they cannot swallow it if they do not), the feed passes into the crop slowly, and is rapidly saturated with the strong, digestive acids of this organ.

It seems to us that this step in the digestive process is entirely overlooked by the advocates of wet mash feeding. It really seems as though the wet mash feeders must consider the crop as only a stopping station, or reservoir, for the food to rest in before passing to the gizzards and intestines. We know that a very important work is performed in the digestive process in the crop, and that the dry feeding method, recognizing this, gets a much higher percentage of efficiency out of the feed, and incidentally, maintains the birds in a much higher standard of health.

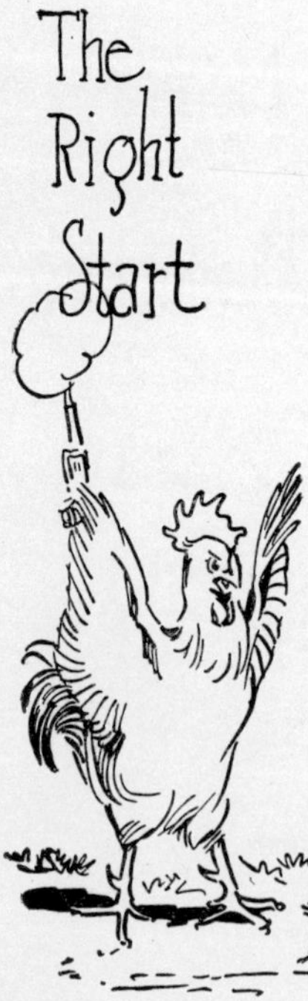

Here the work of digestion is very thoroughly started before the feed passes along the alimentary canal through the intestines, and this supplementary work which Nature intended should be done before the intestines are reached, makes the process much easier and more thorough.

With the newly hatched chicken its destiny is practically made or wrecked during the first three weeks of its existence. If it finds itself

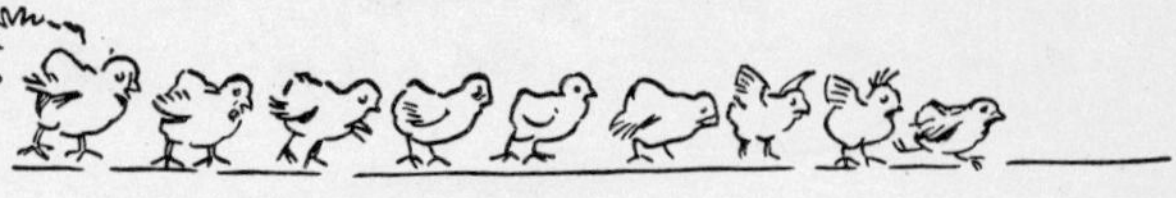

in the land of plenty, with the proper food always within reach, it widens out into a broad gauged chicken, building a digestive system capable of assimilating large quantities of food, and grows into a larger bird than its parents, matures and ripens into one of those wide-tailed, square-bodied, heavy-limbed birds, that are a delight to us all. The pullets are ripe at five or six months of age, and produce eggs plentifully the full year through, and with utter disregard of outside weather conditions.

On the other hand, if the birds are brought up and cared for by one of our skimpy feeders, who thinks that they must be kept hungry all the time, the chickens develop into the thinner stock, who have been taught from infancy to look upon a square meal as a mistake; these mistakes occurring at such rare intervals that the birds cannot accumulate a surplus from which to manufacture eggs. In case a change of ownership gives them the benefit of full feeding, it takes them a long time to get over the shock, and it is a number of weeks especially in the fall of the year, before they get well ripened, matured, and ready to start laying; and they never have the capacity to take in and properly digest the large quantities of food, that is necessary for the most profitable egg production.

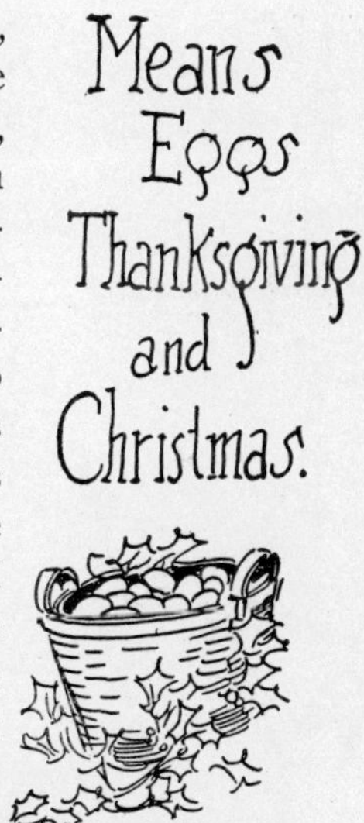

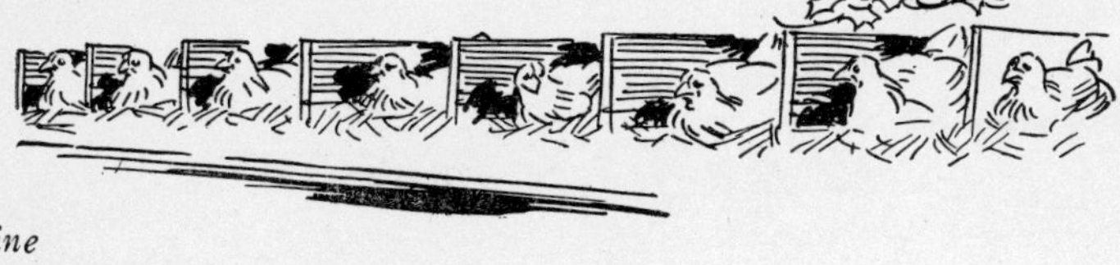

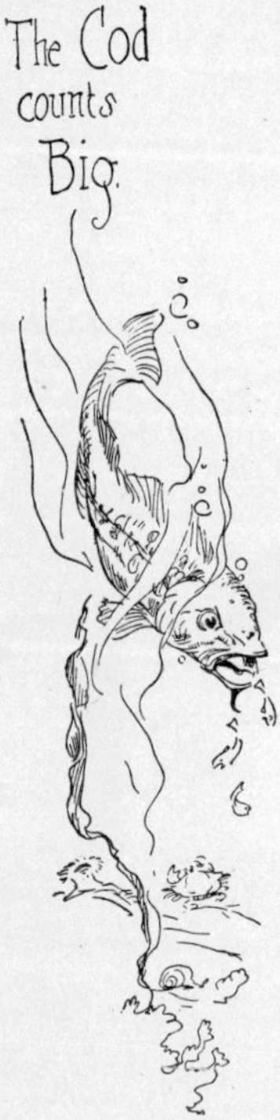

When the chick is first hatched, it has recently absorbed the yolk of the egg in the intestinary chamber, and this furnishes a portion of its food for the next ten days, after which time, in a normally healthy chicken, it disappears.

Now, during this ten-day period, with the yolk to draw on, it is easy to realize that no more animal fat should be added to the ration. But the chickens crave animal food, and grow much better when fed a ration that contains this lean meat, without the fat.

Here again the Cod Fish furnishes just the desired element, and nothing else that we have found answers the purpose. Meat Scraps uniformly contain from 10% to 20% fat.

Going back to the three-weeks-old chickens, let us follow the housing system and general care, aside from the feeding.

Most modern heated brooders are too large for the babies, and too small for the four to six-weeks-old youngsters, unless, as usually occurs, Dame Nature has reduced the flock to one-half or one-third of the original number. The result is crowding in uncomfortable quarters at night, and much loss of efficiency in their general discontent, and much loss to the vitality and economy. Chickens cannot make satisfactory gains when living in bad air, in too small coops, or when suffering from insufficient food or improperly balanced rations, or in too large flocks (one hundred chickens running together and roosting in quarters about right in size for twenty-five chickens).

Twenty-five chickens properly cooped and fed will make as many pounds gain upon one-halr the food consumed, as will fifty chickens improperly housed and fed, and the strangest part of the whole story is that the increased efficiency plan takes no more, in fact takes less, labor than the old plan, and brings much quicker returns. This higher efficiency method gives us full, plump broilers and roasters, ready for market or table at five minutes' notice. The other method gives us broilers and roasters only after a fattening process, two to four weeks behind the other, and from one-half to two pounds less in weight.

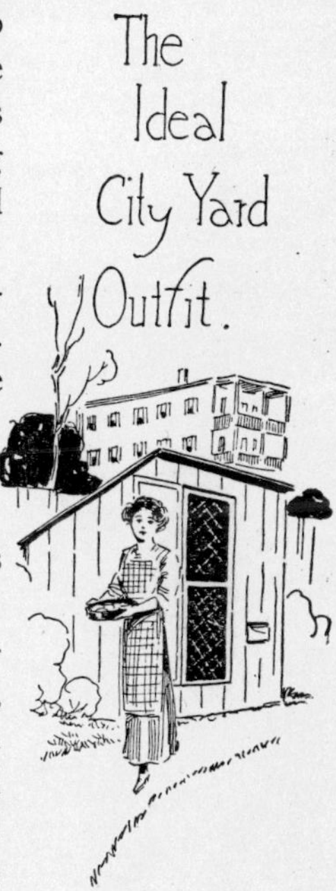

We have taken the chicken through the growing period and marketing age, to the laying pen. From our original three hundred eggs we have ninety to one hundred strong, heavy, well matured efficiency pullets, as against the twenty to thirty-five pullets that matured one to three weeks later, and which were one to two pounds each less in weight on the old plan.

The old style method takes the twenty to thirty-five pullets, places them in a nice warm house, with plenty of glass, feeds them a hot mash in the morning, keeps them more or less suffocated all winter through, reproducing thc same kind of eggs and chickens the following spring; thereby perpetuating the general inefficiency scheme.

The modern higher efficiency plan places these large, well rounded-out pullets in houses costing much less to construct, being one-third or more open to the south, feeds them Egg Feed (before them all the time) and throws Scratch Feed to them once a day. The eggs start early and continue to come all the fall and winter. They hatch out the same kind of high efficiency chickens, and the profits are assured.

These briefly are some of the reasons why the dry feeding system produces so much better results than the old way, and why its users are uniformly successful. A trial of the method will convince you.

Fine for growing and Breeding Stock

The conditions we have portrayed as the results of the old plan actually exist on thousands of poultry plants today. Here and there one owner is considered lucky, while hundreds complain that their birds do not do well, and rail at the tariff, reciprocity, and have a general grouch. Occasionally an owner knows that there must be a reason why every egg fails to hatch, and a reason why every chick dies. He earnestly tries to arrest these troubles, follows our directions, and accepts our statements, and though they seem somewhat radical, has faith, tries them out, and finds even better results than we have predicted.

We are glad to say that thousands of our followers are today much more prosperous from our teachings, but we realize that there are hundreds of thousands yet to be convinced and put upon the higher efficiency plane.

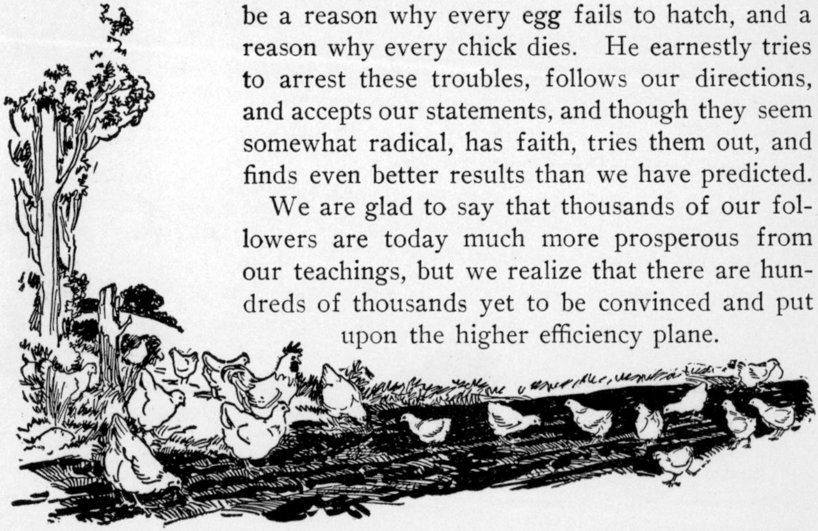

If you have been helped, won't you help your neighbor!

If you are still in the doubting column, won't you make a few tests of these methods, and when convinced hand along your good results, and help spread the good work?

If we all get together we can easily double the poultry crop of the country, and thereby all gain more returns and greater prosperity.

We consider poultry the most profitable crop that can be raised today, and know that the profit now derived from it can be doubled by this system.

There are thousands of families struggling along, striving to make the pay envelope satisfy the butcher and grocery-man, who could keep enough poultry in their back-yard to pay the rent, and at the same time have all the fresh eggs they could eat every morning.

And it does not require a great deal of room at that. A space large enough to set a house 6 x 8 feet in size will do nicely for 15 or 18 hens, on which a profit of from $30 to $50 a year can be easily made, and the outlay need not be over fifty dollars.

Smaller houses and flocks can be started and as much larger as one cares to undertake, but the point is that the thousands who might be

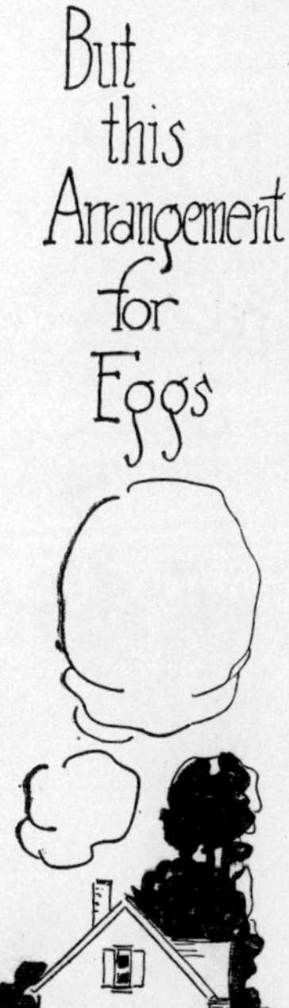

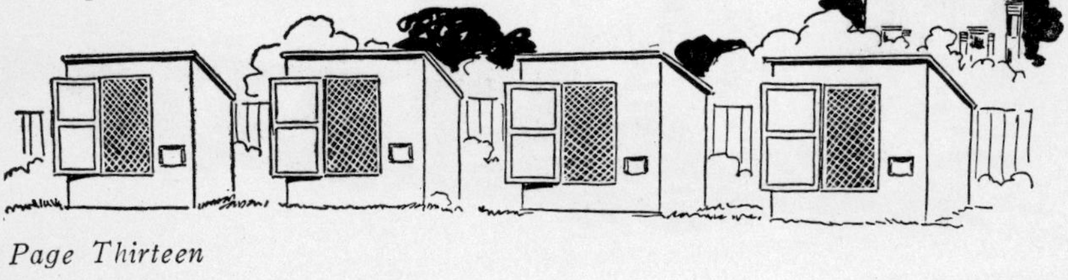

making $50.00 to $300.00 per year right in their own yards are not getting ahead at all.

Look your back-yard over and see if you cannot start. If not, look up another location with back-yard poultry keeping in mind, and then get in on the right basis and get a lead on the grocer.

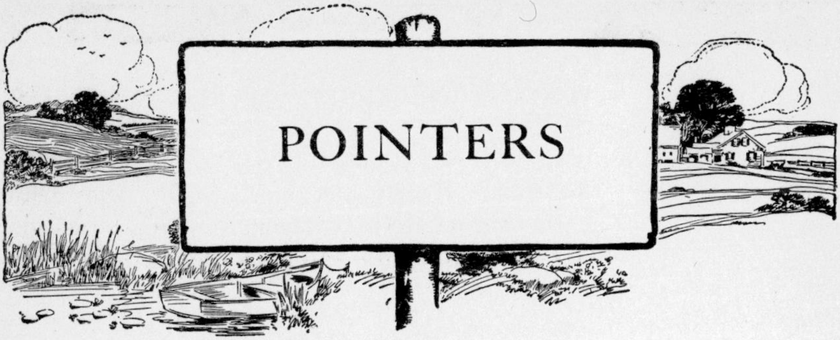

POINTERS

We all admire an artist at his work and it does not matter what that work is, if he is thoroughly efficient.

This work may be painting pictures, rendering musical selections, selling goods, building a house or raising a crop of potatoes or chickens, but so long as he does it better than his competitors or fellow workmen he commands our respect and admiration.

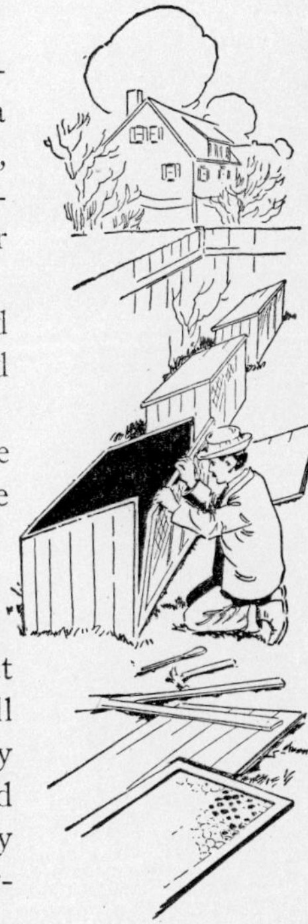

Many times this efficiency will be recognized as doing the right thing at the proper time and in the right place.

In caring for poultry, little things done at the proper time will be found to go to make up the success of a venture.

On the following pages we have attempted to set down the most important of the little things to be looked after each month during that month. To the beginner we know they will prove very helpful in removing needless worry and in simplifying the business. To the old hand at the business they will be found a daily reminder of things that are sometimes overlooked in the stress of the work.

While the chronological order is set for the climate of New England, with slight modifications they will be found to fit almost any climate, giving more air and shade in warmer districts and a little heavier feeding of corn in colder regions, always bearing in mind that when in doubt give the birds more air rather than less.

We hope you will get as much pleasure in following these monthly suggestions as we have in gathering the facts from the pages of experience and setting them down for you.

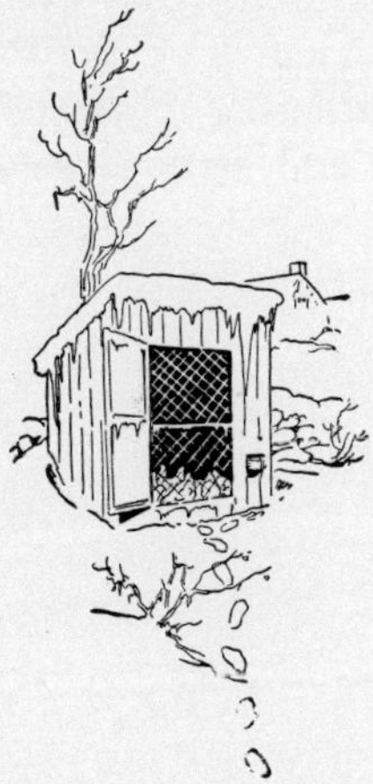

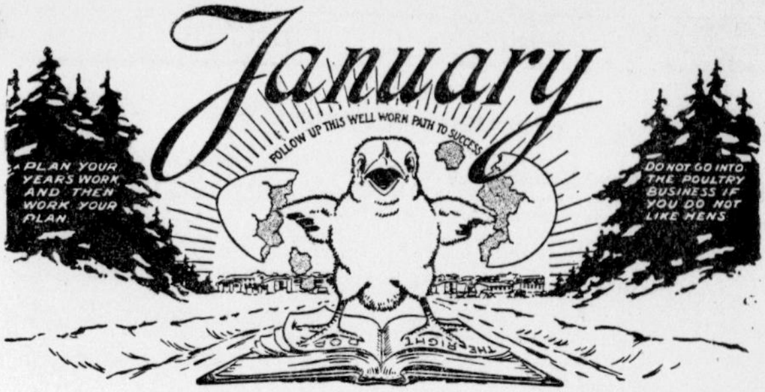

STARTING IN JANUARY

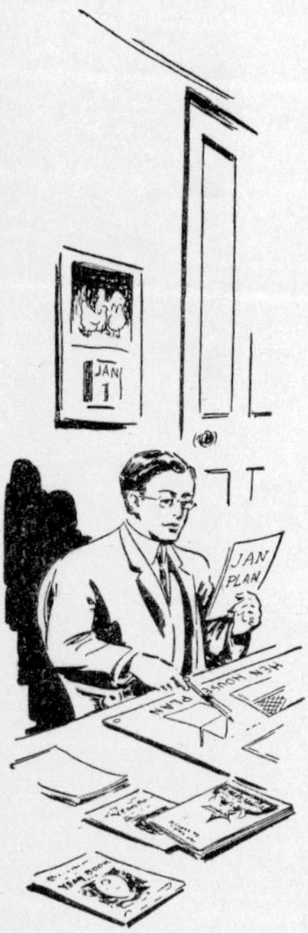

JANUARY is a cold month, but this should not deter any really earnest poultryman from starting in business. Begin by purchasing a portable house along the line of those shown on page 117, or having a similar building constructed. We think in most cases it will be more economical to purchase, but that is for you to decide.

Read carefully housing article on page 117.

We suggest the purchase of 15-18 pullets, with no male bird, if you are in the business to supply your table with fresh eggs alone. If you are starting in to breed your own stock, and this lot is for your original breeding stock, we urge the purchase of not over 10 to 12 females, preferably yearling hens, and a good vigorous cockerel,—one that is well developed and fully up to the standard weight of the variety you have decided shall be your choice. Fill the open stoneware feed dishes with Egg Feed, give them scratch feed once a day, provide fresh water, grit and oyster shells, and you should soon be getting eggs.

Do not go into the poultry business if you do not like hens.

GENERAL SUGGESTIONS

Plan Your Year's Work, and Then Work Your Plan.

January is a good month to plan out the campaign for the next year's or few years' work. Make up your mind, first of all, that you are going to be a high grade poultryman; that you are going to improve your last year's profits; that you are going to raise your stock better this year than you ever did; that you are going to have a plan and stick to it; that nothing will tempt you to keep changing from one breed to another, from raising eggs for market to raising eggs for hatching, from market poultry to fancy poultry; and that you are determined to so improve your breed by careful feeding that they will weigh from one to three pounds more when they go to market, and that the cockerels will go to market from one to two months ahead of any of the neighbors'. You can do it. Stick to it.

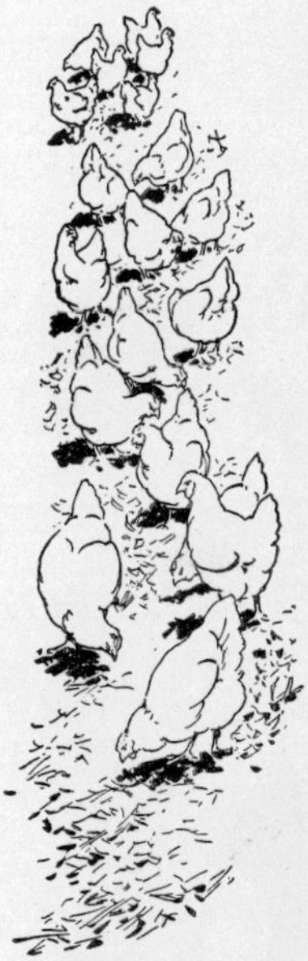

Late hatched June and July pullets should begin laying this month, if they have been properly fed and cared for. Broilers and roasters started this month bring the cream of the year's prices, and the parent stock should be selected as per suggestions in our October and December hints. They should be laying well now, and the incubators and brooders put into working order, and the work started early in the month.

Cut down the number of females in your breeding pens. The annual loss from infertile eggs, weak germs and delicate chickens would total up into millions of dollars. You say that it would be a nuisance to put half as many females in each pen,—well, then, put a partition through each pen. It may be a nuisance, but not half as much as throwing away half of your early hatches.

Small flocks spell big profits, and this rule holds good from start to finish.

The contented hen fills the Egg basket.

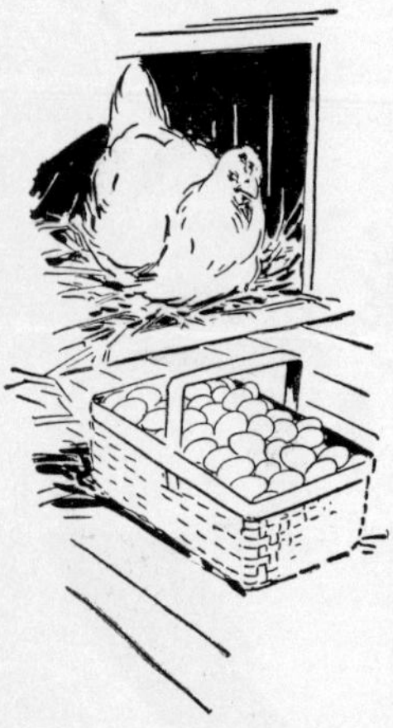

Pampered stock and pampered chicks spell failure.

The contented hen fills the egg basket.

Breeding stock previously selected should be housed in cold houses and fed upon a properly proportioned Egg Feed and scratch feed with oyster shells always within reach. This ration insures a steady egg yield, birds always in good health, and if the stock is such as we have described, eggs are sure to be fertile, and chickens hardy and easily reared. Sloppy, wet-mash, stop-watch feeding is not only nerve racking and continuous drudgery to the owner, but keeps the birds on edge and at all times watching and waiting for the next feed. Where this way is once given a trial, the old methods are sure to be laid on the shelf, and you wonder why this business method was not previously discovered.

Chickens hatched in the middle of winter need good brooding accommodations, and while the style of house and plan of brooder may vary with the owner's fancy, for a safe proposition nothing equals the small colony house with an individual fireless brooder contained therein. The chicks should be kept in the brooders according to directions until one week or ten days old, then allowed the run of the dirt floor of the house for another week.

When two weeks old daily out-of-door exercise must be provided and insisted upon. Chickens cannot grow successfully without it, and leg weakness is sure to follow if one attempts to rear them without this. Feed them something they like on a bare spot of ground just outside the building, and provide easy access to and from the house (no stairs or blind passageway) and they will work back and forth under zero weather conditions with nothing but benefit to themselves and their owner.

Baled shavings make excellent litter. Most grain dealers carry it in stock.

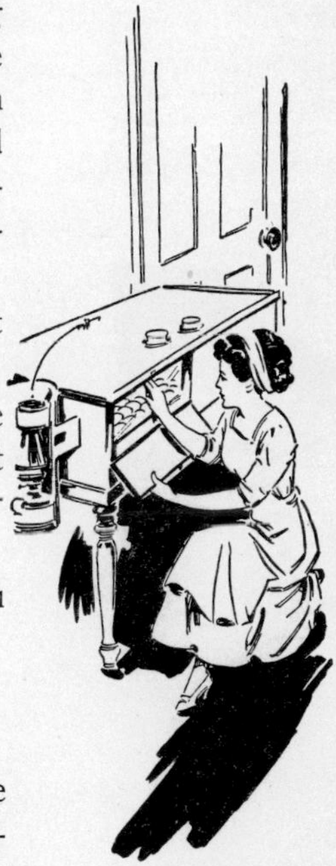

Better give the breeding hens a little more room than the layers, and if you find you must sell a few pullets in order to do this, ask your live poultry dealer to quote.

Get your incubator this month and be sure you have plenty of brooding room.

JANUARY DISEASES

The only trouble for January, and most of the fall and early winter months, is roup—or neglected colds, caused usually by crowded sleeping quarters, or roosting in draughts or in too warm houses without sufficient air.

Birds housed in houses that are one-third open to the weather on the south side, (or more open in southern climates), will be free from roup or colds if the opening allows no draught. It is the safest way.

To AVOID DRAUGHTS, long houses must have tight board partitions between each pen. Colony houses should be fairly tight on all sides, but the south, and the opening here should be about two feet from the floor, and sides and roof as illustrated by cut of "No-Yard" house on page 28.

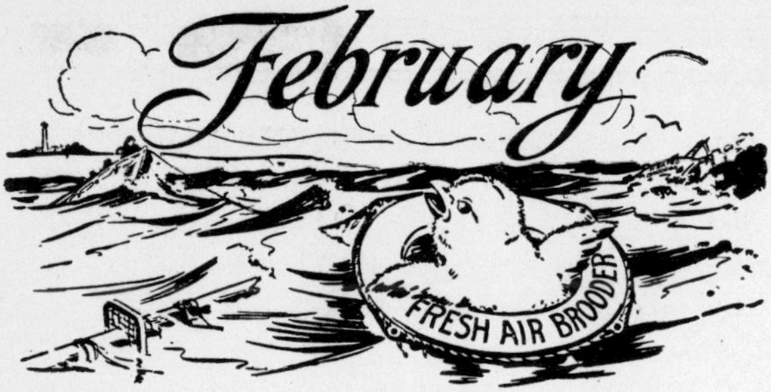

STARTING IN FEBRUARY

THE conditions for starting the poultry business in February are much the same as for January, except that for breeding purposes it is easier to procure well developed pullets that will make satisfactory breeders, although stronger chickens will be the rule if yearlings are used as recommended for January. Get an incubator, if raising chickens is your object, and start it up as soon as the eggs come freely.

Our cities are growing rapidly; our people are appreciating the value of fresh eggs. The price keeps working up and will continue to work up until you receive 75c. per dozen for eggs during the holidays. Get aboard!

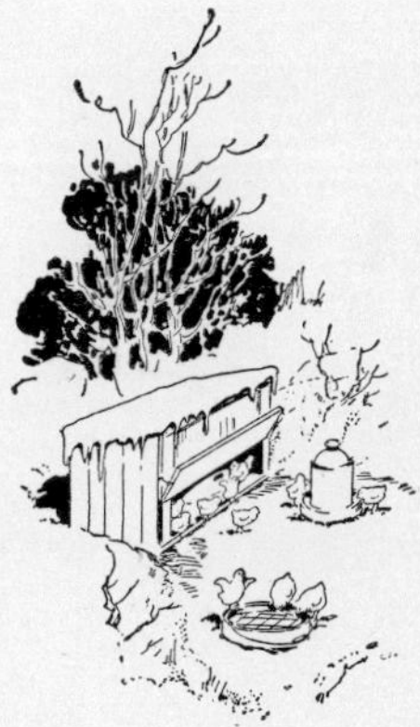

Do not spend much money on fancy breeds, new varieties, and new blood. If you will take proper care of your own stock, you can develop it into as good and hardy a stock, and handsome as any you see in the show rooms.

Keep your expenses and your ideas down to the market level of price, and you will make money, while if you try for the long prices of fancy stock, you will find only disappointment and loss.

We have been there,—we have won the ribbons, and sold the high priced birds,—but take it from us, THERE IS NOTHING IN IT. It is the good market biddy that has no frills, fancy skirts or shirtwaists, that pays the grocery bills and the mortgage.

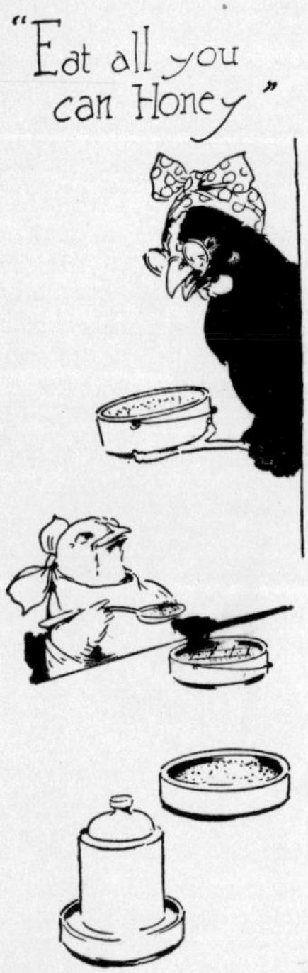

GENERAL SUGGESTIONS

Winter chickens, in fact all chickens, should be well fed in order to get the benefit of the quick-growing habit of the previously selected ancestors. Surely the youngsters cannot make bone and muscle out of a "pleasant view" or "good sunny weather;" something more satisfying to the appetite will answer much better, and while plenty of good vitalizing air must be provided, so must an abundance of food be always within reach.

Use plenty of good litter. The birds need exercise to keep in the condition that means profitable poultry.

Keep the Egg Feed hopper full. The birds are keeping union hours now.

Scald out the drinking dishes occasionally.

If your early hatches show signs of leg weakness, be sure that you get them an out-of-door run. In fact, feed them out of doors on the bare ground one or two feeds per day of some delicacy that they are very fond of. Get them out into the open air after they are ten days of age regardless of temperature. Shovel off a spot right down to mother earth, and do not be afraid to let them eat a little snow. Place your orders now for baby chickens for April delivery.

You will have to put on your thinking cap often nowadays, or the other spring work will crowd out the chicks. Do the fair thing by them. Their success during the rest of the year depends on it.

Chicks of the large American breeds hatched this month will make the best of early roasters, and will bring good prices in June and July.

Start the brooder in a clean house, with not more than 25 chicks together; feed chick feed liberally, better up to the wasting point than to let some of the chicks go hungry. Start the Growing Feed as soon as they are one week old, and let them have the run of the house when ten days old. Do not let them bunch up out in the bright sunlight on cold winter days. The sunlight has a fascination for them and frequently they will huddle together and get chilled outside in preference to going to a warm hover chamber. In wooden brooders it is sometimes better to hang a thin curtain over the glass window to avoid this trouble, until they reach a more discriminating age.

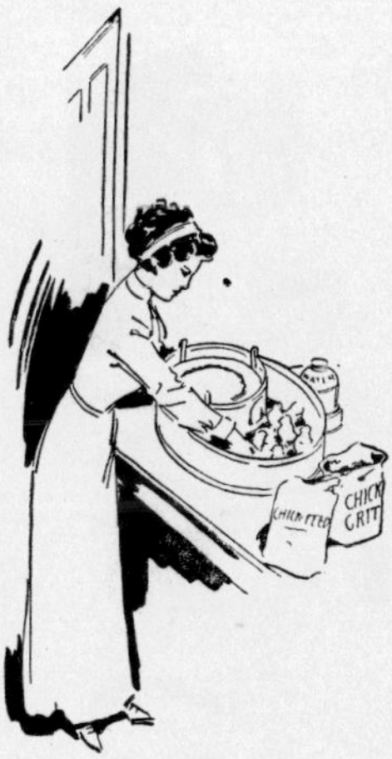

If your rooster is old, do not have too many hens in the pen with him, if you expect the eggs to hatch.

If one keeps hens for egg production alone, there will be no need of having any male birds. It costs at least $1.00 a year to feed a male. Better keep an extra hen.

FEBRUARY DISEASES

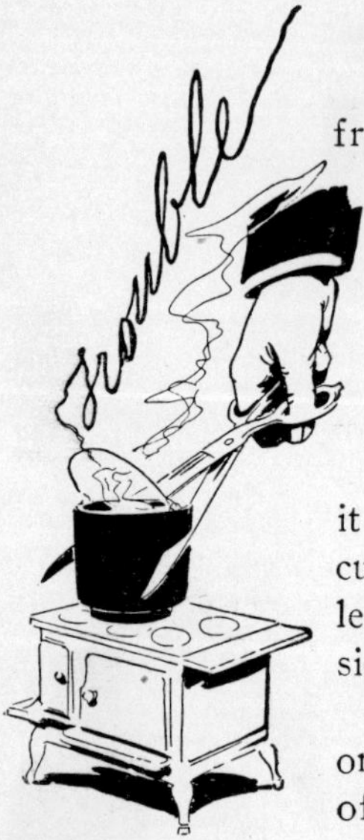

Cut out the hot
Mash
It spells TROUBLE

This month's troubles, if any, are likely to be from confinement, sometimes resulting in egg eating and feather pulling, caused by the birds not getting all the variety of feed which they pick up while on range.

These elements should be supplied in the Egg Feed, thereby eliminating all chances of this trouble.

Canker sometimes appears this month, but it is really a case of roup that you thought you cured last fall. Healthy hens do not have it unless they drink out of the same dish with the sick ones.

MORAL: Isolate or dispose of all doubtful ones, and continue the isolation until you dispose of them.

Crop bound birds have not been getting enough roughage in their food, and to satisfy the craving, eat their litter, straw or long hay used in making nests. This long material accumulates in the crop, and sometimes causes death.

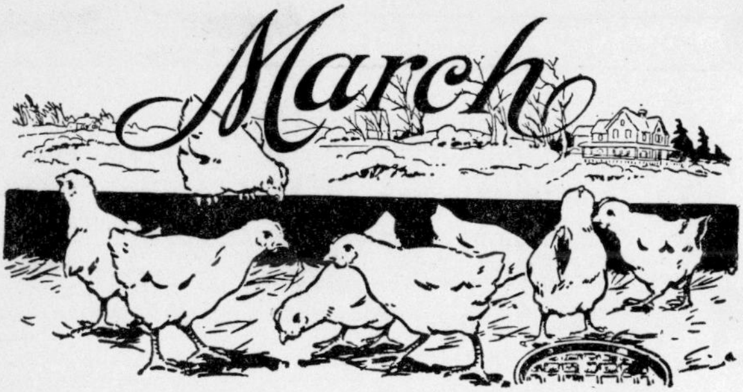

STARTING IN MARCH

CARRY out the January plan and directions on page 121 as to getting the house ready and setting it up; except that starting with newly hatched chickens no litter would be required. This is a very good plan if economy on first cost is the object.

This house makes a fine brooding house for two small brooders and fifty chickens, using the dropping board on which to handle the brooders until the chicks are a week or ten days old,—then giving them the use of the house, separating the two lots with a little chicken wire. When two weeks old provide runways outside, covered to keep out the cats, and when the cockerels are ready for broilers, ship them alive to market, giving the pullets the entire house in which to mature.

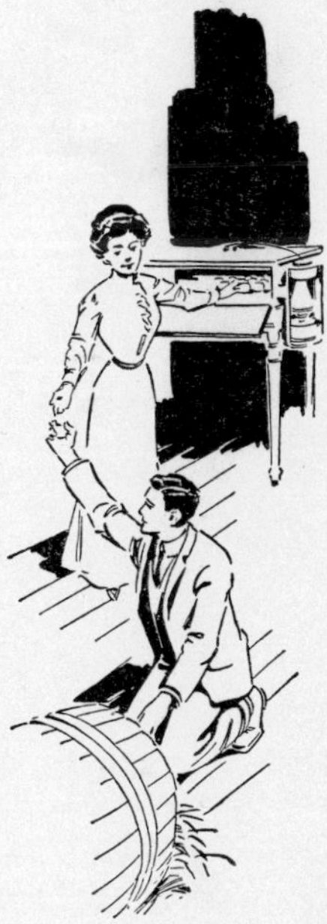

While this plan does not provide an immediate income, it costs very little to start it, and the cockerels sold should pay for the feed that they and the pullets have consumed up to date.

Do not go into the poultry business if you think you can half feed your flock and make a success of the business. The hen's body wants come first; if there is any surplus it is made up into eggs. It is up to you to provide the surplus.

GENERAL SUGGESTIONS

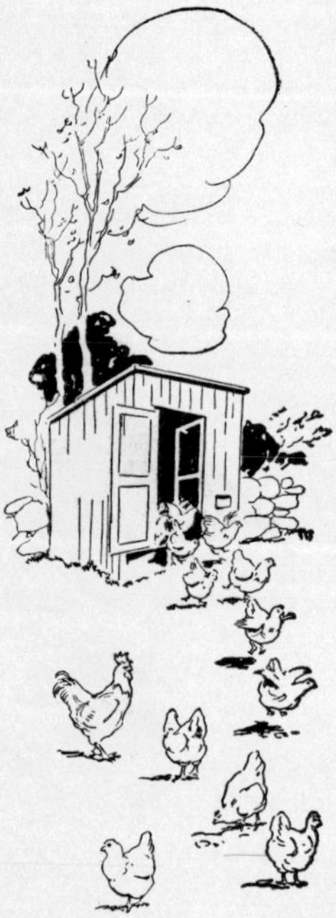

When planning your extensions for the year, if you build your roosting coops for your young stock on the colony laying house plan, you will find that your capital is working twelve months in the year; whereas, if you use a low, small roosting coop, you must rebuild again in the fall. Select a type of colony house that pleases you, then add to your plant each season as many of these colony houses or units, as you need.

Brains are needed as much as capital in the poultry business.

Following a hard winter, this is the month of poor hatches from stock that has been fed upon wet mashes and partially smothered all winter in glass houses. Such stock needs a few weeks' exercise in the open air to get thoroughly alive again.

Set all the broody hens that come along this month.

Keep the incubator full. After ten days swap the eggs out from under the hens into the incubator. The machine will finish them up better than the hens and deliver more chickens, *with no lice.* An incubator and the hens working together make a splendid combination, and beats either one working alone.

Healthy chickens live unless abused. Healthy hens lay eggs, that if not abused, hatch healthy chickens. Now it is up to you; if you are losing chickens, why? Are you abusing them, or did you abuse the old stock? Abuse may come in two forms,—neglect or over-attention,—trying to keep your birds too warm in winter, feeding improper feeds, etc. You may be keeping your chicks too warm, not running your incubator properly. There is a reason for the death of every chicken. Try and see this year if you cannot cut last season's mortality one-half.

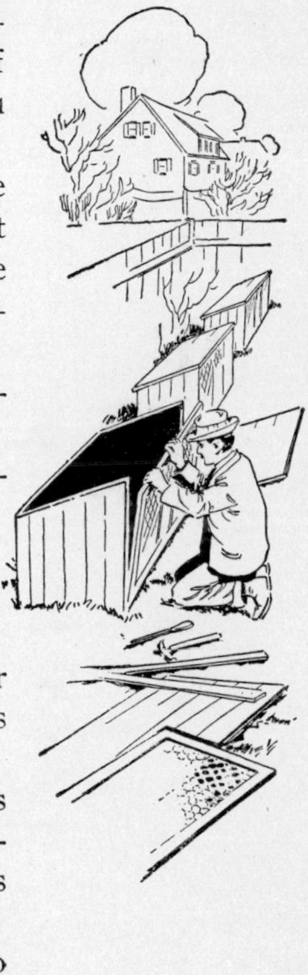

Early January hatched broilers can now be marketed, as the demand for this month does not call for them to weigh over three-quarters to one pound each. Market limited as to number required.

Pullets hatched this month will give good results in the fall.

Cockerels of the American varieties, March-hatched, caponized, sell at good prices for roasting chickens during August and early September. This month is usually the year's lowest point for prices on eggs.

Alfalfa cut or mealed makes splendid litter for brooders and runs for early chicks, always sweet and not expensive.

Figure out about how many broods of chicks there will be, and get the spring coops and fittings cleaned up and in working order. Chickens will soon be plenty, and time scarce.

In mating the pens of breeding stock refer to October hints for the selection of male birds, and December hints on the selection of females. Remember that nothing but the best is good enough, whether for eggs, roasters, broilers or fancy poultry.

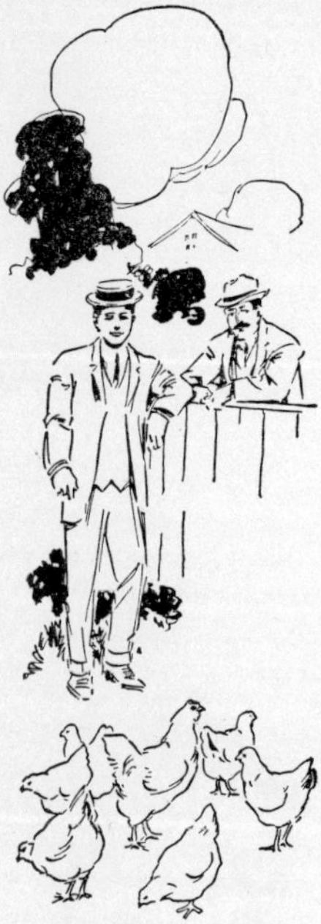

Tell your neighbor about your success

MARCH DISEASES

Leg weakness in chickens is caused usually by confining the birds indoors, and on hard floors and overheated brooders. Get your birds out of doors when ten days old, and raise them always (all of them) in small heatless brooders.

Sitting hens leave their nests if lousey—seldom for any other reason. Use lice powder liberally whenever you set a hen, and at other times also.

Poor fertility is usually caused by insufficient air in the quarters during the winter, too many females with one male, or too large flocks. Cut down the size of your flocks, and take out the windows, substituting wire netting, water-proof sheeting, or cheese cloth.

Raise your chickens on a new lot of land each season, or let a crop of green stuff grow between seasons, and you will not be troubled with gapes in your chicks.

April

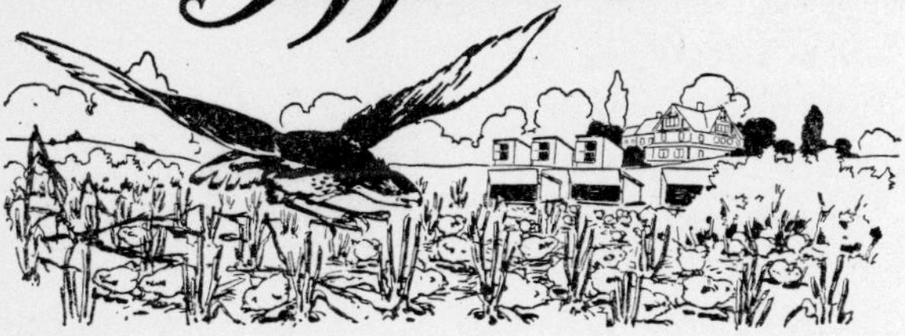

STARTING IN APRIL

Starting in April is a cinch. Buy the houses as in January plan, and if eggs for table is all that is wanted, you will not have long to wait. Your pullets will be laying within a day or two after you get them, and in a week's time you will be getting a dozen eggs or more a day.

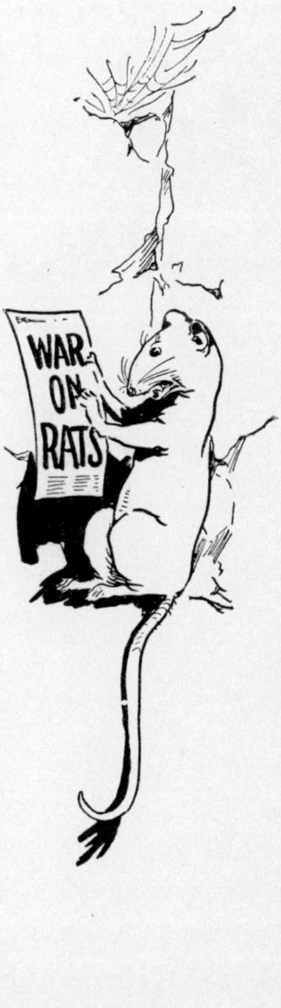

If you wish to start with the minimum expense and are willing to wait for the chickens to grow, get a small portable house and two small heatless brooders and proceed as in March using the house for the pullets after the cockerels go to market.

Using incubators, you simply provide more small brooders as the chickens hatch.

If hatching with hens, set them in a dry place with plenty of ventilation. Avoid damp cellars. Forget about sods and damp earth in the nest.

GENERAL SUGGESTIONS

If your chickens are on range or in yards where the hawks bother them, sometimes convenient brush heaps, or stretches of wire netting, so placed as to break up the swoop of the hawks as they skim along the ground in catching the chickens, will stop their thieving.

In early spring a cornfield, with last season's stalks standing, makes an ideal dodging place for the youngsters, and Mr. Hawk will give it up as a "bad job" trying to catch them among the stalks.

There is only one way to feed poultry if you would make a success of the business; stuff them with the right kind of feed from "hatch to hatchet."

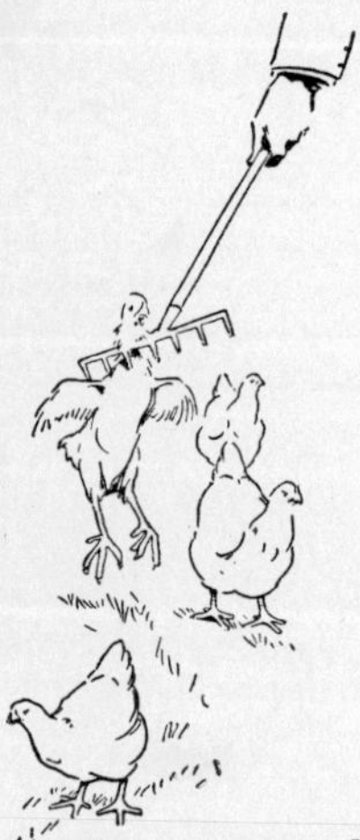

Weed out the Long Legs

Watch the cockerels and pullets, and mark now the ones making the most satisfactory growth, choosing those that have grown steadily and at all times have been plump, full breasted, and in good proportion.

Avoid those that grow leggy, with thin breasts, and also the ones that grow unevenly, making a month's or two months' progress and then apparently stopping, and later going ahead again.

Get the breeding stock out of doors, give them plenty of room, not too many females with your males.

If you have previously lacked the nerve, take all the windows out of your poultry house this month, provided, of course, that they are all in the south side and no draughts on the roost results.

Growing Feed is the feed that puts those nice plump broilers and roasters on the market, and gives us the big hardy pullet that lays all winter, and in the spring produces the kind of chicks that are bound to live if given half a chance—and proper feeds.

Cull your flock closely. Market everything that is not making valuable use of every kernel of grain it eats. Do not house any loafers. Get them into money.

Your late chickens will still be in danger from rats. Be sure to keep some good Rat Destroyer in stock and use promptly.

Do not be afraid to give the chicks all the sour milk they will *eat*. Good for them. If there is anything better, we have never found it.

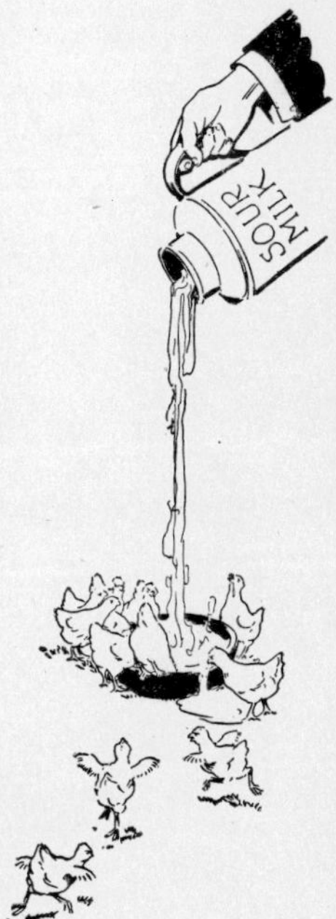

Better caponize the cockerels if intended for roasters. Place in fair sized yards or let them run at large, and feed—*and feed hard.* These chickens are going to be worth thirty cents a pound in June and you cannot afford to have them stand around a minute waiting for the feed to come.

Try this year and have a nice lot of 5 or 6 pound soft roasting chickens to sell during the Christmas holidays.

Use all the poultry manure in top-dressing the grass land or on the garden plot.

January and February hatched broilers are now selling well, and prices during this month should be at the top. If you think there is more money in them for you as broilers, let them go now, if they are large enough. The market calls for larger broilers this month than in February and March, and wants still larger sizes in May. Always give the party paying the bill what they want—if they call for two pound broilers, do not send them one and one-quarter pound, or you will lose in price.

25 Hatched

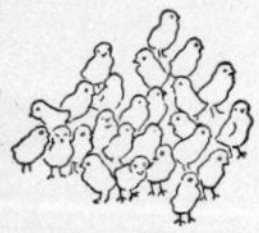

23 Half Grown

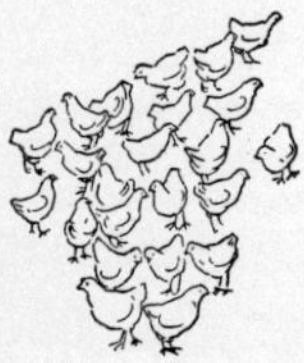

22 Reach maturity

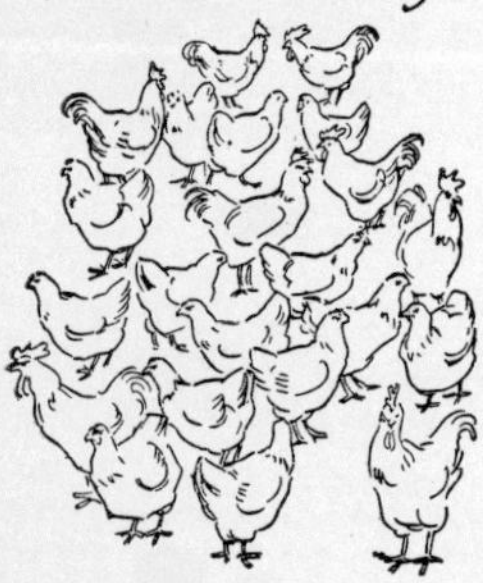

This is one of the best months to hatch pullets for middle-fall and early winter laying. Get out all you can.

Do not throw away that setting of eggs simply because the hen left the nest and they got cold. Unless they have been exposed to freezing temperature for 24 hours, in many instances the hatch will come along as if nothing had happened, if you put another hen on and let her finish the clutch.

Get away from the old idea that you should keep fifty chickens in a lot. You will make almost, if not quite as much profit on twenty-five chickens raised in the small heatless brooder as with fifty raised in the old-fashioned way.

APRIL DISEASES

As a rule poor hatches are the result of low vitality in the breeding stock. (See March hints referring to poor fertility).

Liver troubles and indigestion are caused by poor food and improperly balanced rations.

Guard against these by feeding only the best of feeds.

Chicken pox is some more of last fall's cured (?) colds and roup, now showing up in another form.

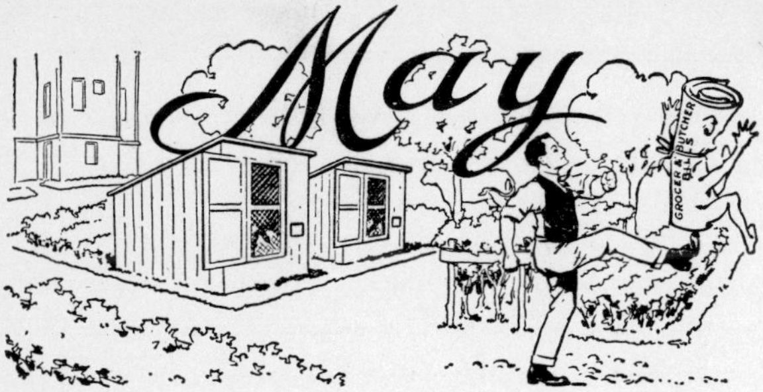

STARTING IN MAY

PULLETS for laying or breeding had better be the rule for starting in May. Set the house up and raise the chickens, if that is to be the business, in the small brooder; or start as in April. The house will soon be needed, and makes an ideal roosting coop. Use the incubator and brooder if you are breeding your own stock.

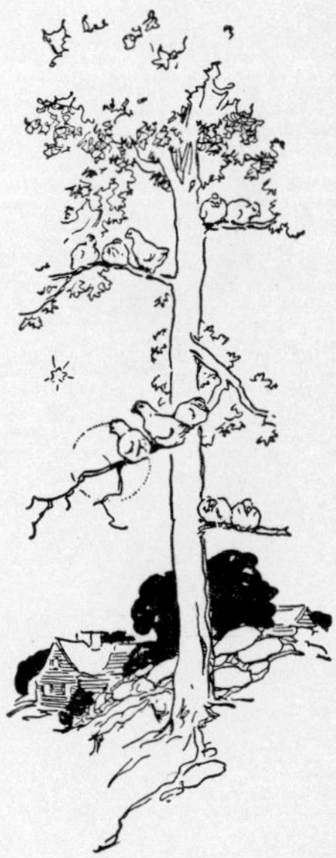

GENERAL SUGGESTIONS

A good garden, a cow, a flock of hens, and you can cut your grocery and provision bill in half and begin to live where you only existed before.

Let the March chickens have plenty of roomy roosting coops or roost in trees. Keep the feed always within reach.

To break up your setting hens, catch them the first night you find them on the nest, and place them in light airy coops, with wire or slat bottoms. This kind of a coop keeps them from hugging a board floor or the ground, and by permitting the free circulation of air below them, tends to reduce the fever which is in their blood at this time.

Lice Spoiled This Hatch

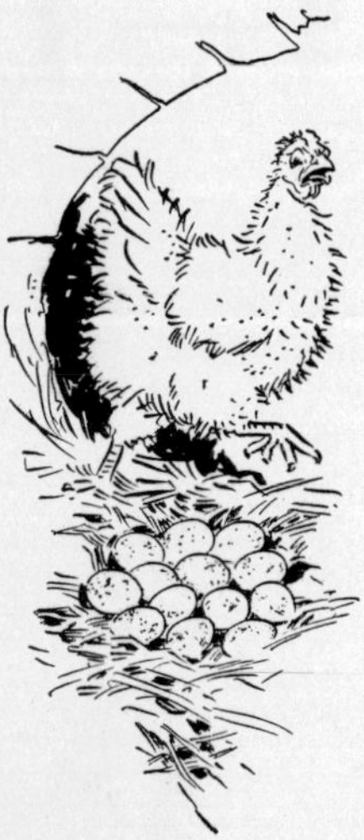

Nothing but lice will cause the old hen to leave her eggs when she has settled down.

Setting hens are lice breeders. This is one reason why the incubator is to be preferred for hatching chickens.

The chickens are free from lice to begin with and it is not such a difficult matter to keep the lice in subjection.

Stop the red mites with liquid lice killer before they get started—prevention is better than cure.

Hatch the eggs in an incubator or with hens.

Don't have ventilators.

Don't try to keep your birds warm. They have ample protection from the coldest winter weather if you only keep them cold all the time.

Don't feed hot mashes that will sweat them.

Keep them healthy, feed them properly, and the eggs will roll out.

Try marketing your birds alive. We don't know of a more nerve-racking job than picking a lot of broilers without tearing the skins.

Many times you can get as much for them alive as you can for them dressed. The labor saved is a big item.

Broilers are going down in price, and the market is calling for larger birds, two and one-half to three pounds each month.

March hatched chickens should now be leaving the brooders, and if they have been properly hardened, will take quite airy roosting coops.

Chicks of the Plymouth Rock, Wyandotte, R. I. Red and some other varieties hatched this month can be brought to laying by November

1st, if pushed with plenty of Growing Feed.

Outdoor brooders must be kept under a shed or some kind of sun protection to maintain the even hover temperature desired. In teaching young chickens to run in and out of outdoor brooders regularly, use a sod or pile of dirt for them to run up and down on. Also when building their first yards make them A-shaped, with the apex at the opening of the brooder, then the chicks will have no corner to bunch up in during the bright sunshiny days, and their education takes much less of the attendant's time.

Growing chickens in the hot months, too young to roost, will thrive much better if they sit on the ground; that is, if their coops have no floors.

Plant Dwarf Essex Rape this month. Care for it as you would young cabbage plants, until the plants are a foot high, then break or cut off the leaves as wanted daily for the poultry. The new shoot will spring up again and continue the process until the hard freezing weather of October and November comes. Four pounds of seed, for an acre of land.

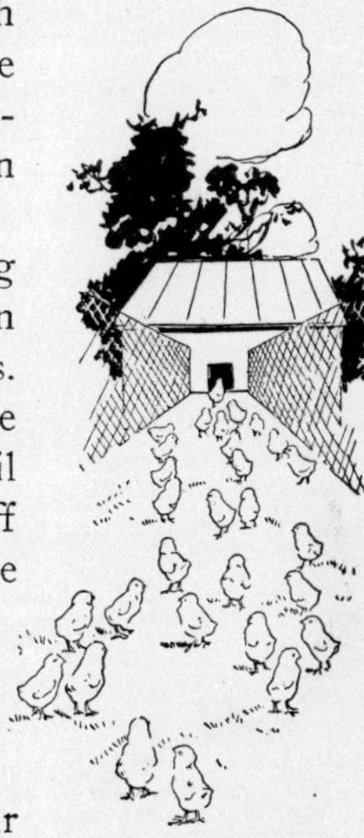

All headed to the Hole

If you are through hatching, break up your pens and market the old cocks, all but the very choice ones that you are expecting to use another year. They are a nuisance with their quarrelsome habits and are a continual bill of expense.

Be liberal enough with your estimate and have chickens enough and to spare. If you have twenty-five percent to spare when filling your laying houses they will always find a ready sale, and this gives you an opportunity to cull

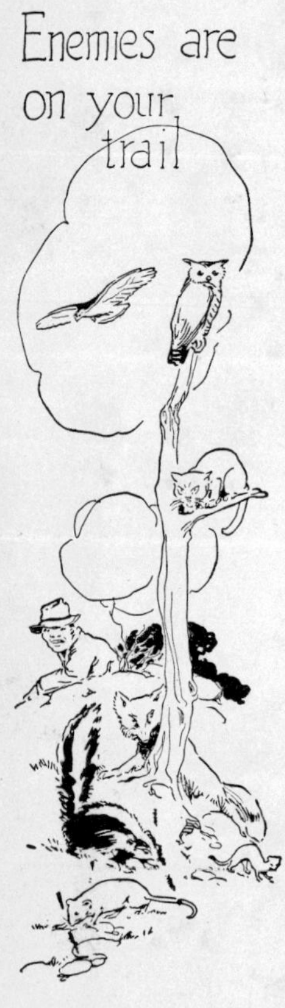

closely and reserve only the best for yourself.

Be careful of them on cool nights when first put out; see that they do not pile up and smother one another.

January and February chickens intended for early market should have grass runs and Growing Feed before them during the balance of their lives.

Have a closely woven wire door to each of your chicken houses and don't forget to close them at night, or some rat, skunk, owl, fox, cat, mink or weasel may deplete your stock.

MAY DISEASES

White diarrhœa is quite contagious among the newly hatched chickens. Raise them in heatless brooders and burn the brooder if any trouble appears.

We think this is an inherited disease. Don't breed from any hens that are not in the best of health and be careful where you buy eggs for hatching.

Be sure you know that any stock you buy is better in health than your own before you part with any of your good money.

We should take chances with a little inbreeding from strong, robust, hardy stock, rather than take chances with unknown, over-advertised outsiders.

If your hens have pale combs look for red mites or spider lice in cracks and all around the roosts and nest boxes. Use liquid lice killer.

Indigestion—See April hints on Liver Troubles.

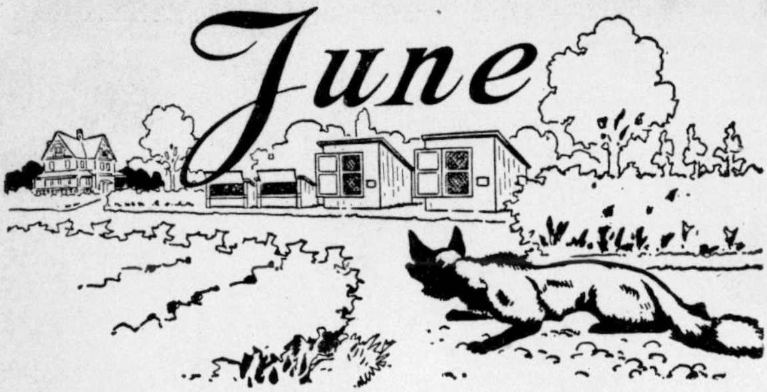

STARTING IN JUNE

STARTING in June, if you want winter laying, it will save time to purchase chickens in place of hatching them. Get them out on a good grass plot with shade and sunlight where they can get whichever they choose when they reach the age of discrimination, and feed liberally. They should be laying in December if pushed with liberal feeding.

Eggs for the family table come as soon as the pullets are located and get to eating freely. Give them all the table scraps after each meal.

GENERAL SUGGESTIONS

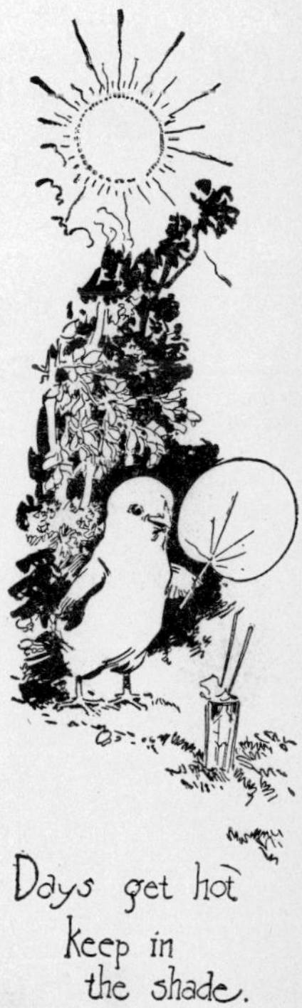

The days begin to get hot; see that the brooders are in the shade, that the chickens have shade also, that they all have an abundance of water and green food. Both are cheap and almost equally important. One-third of the growing chicks living will be from green food if given a grass run, and how much cheaper the gain on this ration is easily figured.

Whitewash the chicken coops. Disinfect the hen houses with a good disinfectant at least once a week, and continue through the hot months to come.

When dressing poultry be careful to cool the carcass properly, else it will heat and result in loss. "Cool well, keep well," is the rule.

From June 1st to July 4th is the top of the market for roasting chickens. January and February roasters, capons and pullets should all be turned into money while the price is at the highest point. They should bring from 30c. to 33c. per pound, and here is where we think the roaster has great advantage over the broiler. These same chickens in April were broiler size, and would not have sold for a great deal more per pound that month and were weighing only two pounds each. They now weigh four to five pounds each, and the last two or three pounds have only cost eight to ten cents per pound for feed, giving a profit of from twenty to twenty-five cents per pound, or from forty to seventy-five cents per bird. No mortality and a handsome margin.

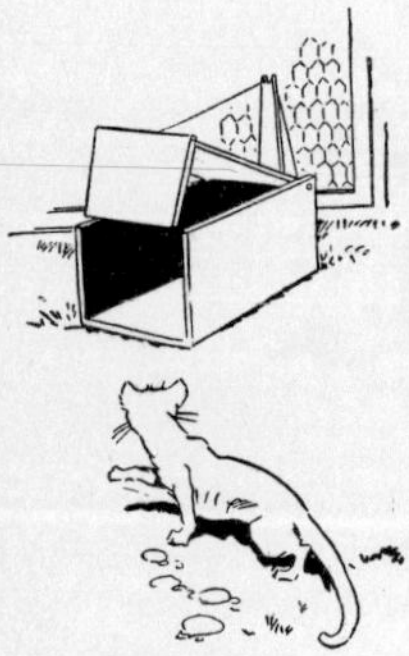

A good suggestion for stray cats.

Look hard after lice and use liquid lice killer and lice powder freely. Don't let the "bugs" get a start.

Cats and chickens agree sometimes, but stray cats are always subject to suspicion and if you are losing chickens and can trace them in no other way, set a box trap, and bait it with a dead chicken. If the cat takes the bait, your suspicion is correct. Dispose of the cat with as little delay and disturbance as possible.

A box trap is made of boards and illustrated below. Most any boy that is handy with tools will make one in an hour or two and most country boys have used them to catch rabbits and other game. They need no directions or suggestions.

Remove males from breeding yards as soon as the season is over. Keep the best for another season. If you have three or four, put all together in an open yard on a good hot day at noon time and let them "scrap it out." In a few minutes they will find the master, and all future disputes will be referred to him for settlement. Keep them by themselves until wanted for breeding pens.

Begin to work off the less valuable and more broody of the hens.

This is a good month to caponize.

Market all the broiler stock on hand.

Have you provided shade in the runs? Failure to do so results in chicks that won't feather.

Get the layers to drink all the water or milk you can. Eggs are very largely made up of water, and the birds cannot lay heavily without a constant supply. Frequent changes induce frequent drinking.

Milk, (skimmed, sweet or sour) is one of the best feeds for growing chickens and it will pay double the profit when turned into poultry that it will when fed to pigs.

If you want to use brooding hens, this and next month are good months to set them.

They will raise a greater percentage of chicks during the hot weather than brooders, and, if allowed to take their own course, will raise these and go to laying again during August and September, when eggs are paying a good profit.

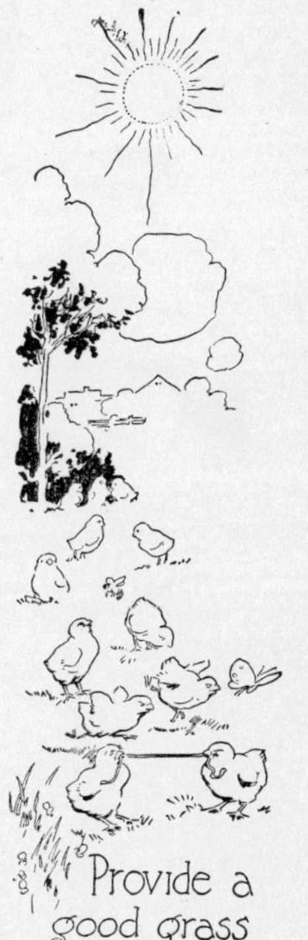

We have no use for the hen in hatching during the cold weather, but she will be found to do good work during the hot months in brooding chickens. Give her a corn field, orchard or patch of weeds in which to grow her family, and she will nearly pay for herself before cold weather gets her.

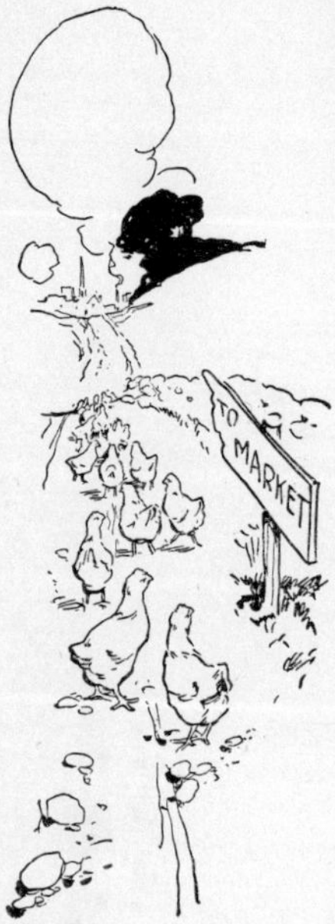

JUNE DISEASES

Sudden deaths during hot weather are many times the result of last fall's cured (?) cases of roup.

The Barred Rocks seem a little more prone to these troubles than other varieties.

Late chicks not growing is usually the result of carelessness, unclean brooders, or yarding them in the same yards the early chicks used, or from mixing the young and older chickens together.

Be sure to keep each age by themselves, and be just as enthusiastically clean with these late comers as with your first born pets that came in March.

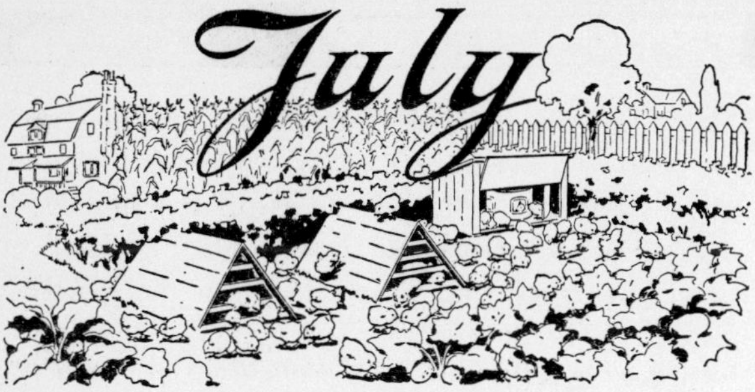

STARTING IN JULY

Starting this month we should purchase large heavy pullets if for the table eggs alone, depending upon using them upon the family table during the months of August and September, when they begin moulting. It is rather late to hatch breeding stock for another year. We would advise purchasing chickens and pushing them along so they would get to laying in January. This can be easily done if new runs, plenty of shade, feed and green stuff are provided.

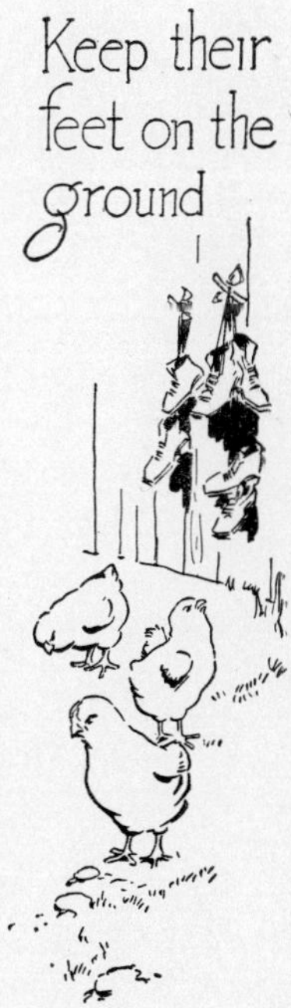

GENERAL SUGGESTIONS

If you will see that all your chickens that are not old enough to perch sit with their feet on the ground during the hot weather, you will avoid colds and roup among them.

There is a wonderful amount of blood passing through their feet, and if the ball of the foot rests upon the ground (the earth being a remarkably good conductor of heat) this keeps their body temperature down, and prevents sweating and consequent colds.

Board floors are necessary in the early spring months to keep the coops dry, and are decidedly wrong in hot weather, for the above reasons.

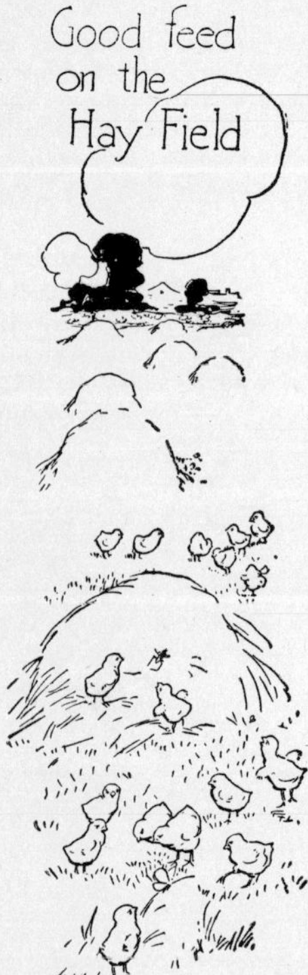

The demand is for heavy chickens and heavy fowl.

Spread the growing youngsters out over the hay fields this month after the hay is cut and you will lose nothing, next season's crop will be better for it, and if you lose some of the second crop it will be fed to better advantage to the chickens than to any other farm animals.

Do not think that the chickens can live on grasshoppers; give them all the feed you can get them to eat, with the grasshoppers as an extra.

After this season of the year it is a good thing to send broody hens to market.

July is termed a late month for hatching laying pullets, but if you have not ample stock, by all means get out enough to "make good." If these chickens are given as good care as outlined for June chicks, they will mature in January and February and make the best of summer and early fall layers. It is useless to expect the early hatched pullet to keep laying all winter and spring and still keep at it through the hot weather. Really, these late pullets are nearly or quite as profitable as the earlier ones, for they lay splendidly during August, September and October, when fresh eggs bring good prices and at a very small cost. Do not despise the late chickens.

About this time put the caponized males in yards fifty feet square for fifty birds, push them with fattening feed and plenty of meat scraps, with liberal feeds of corn and barley. Do not hold them too long. When they reach the weight of 5 lbs. each alive, get market quotations. Remember, as a general thing, the price per pound is going down after they reach this size, and it is up to you to get your money out of them at the earliest opportunity.

For instance, a 5-pound chicken sold in August will usually bring 18 to 20 cents per pound, while if the same cockerel is kept until November, then weighing 6 pounds, he will be hard and not worth 12 to 15 cents per pound. In other words, you have lost three months' feeding by holding.

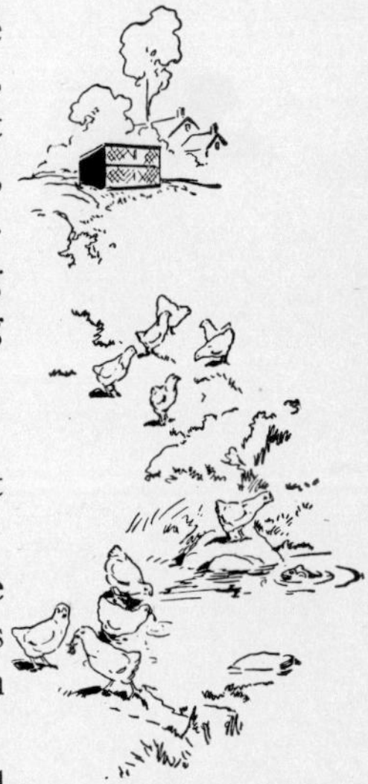

Allow chicks the run of swamp land during hot weather, but get them into upland brooding coops at night or colds may result.

Keep the house as cool as possible.

The most profitable hens, as a rule, are not the stylish ones.

Lice like to hide away under the end of the roosts. Every time you spray, lift the roosts and give the pests a dose that will drive them out for good and all.

Women make the best of poultry keepers and all find the work interesting, pleasant and very profitable.

There ought to be a law forbidding over twenty-five chicks together.

Renew the nest material frequently.

Send the broilers to market as fast as they are ready. Write your dealer for quotations and get them into money, giving the pullets more room.

Look out for mites in all your new coops and houses as well as in the old ones, but they seem to thrive better in the old wood. Use liquid lice killer all around cracks, nests and roosts of laying houses and roosting coops.

Shady nooks are relished by the hens.

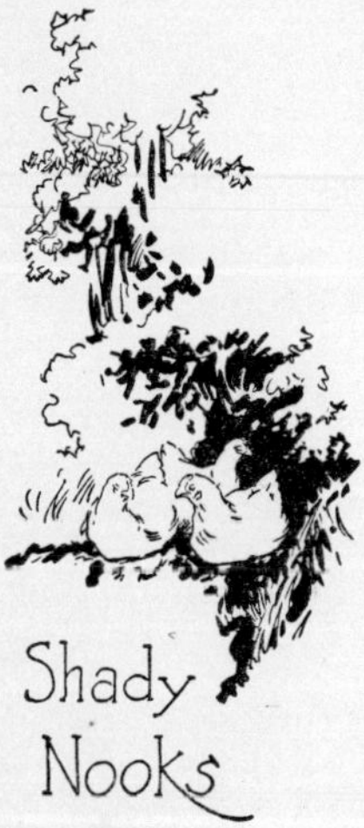

JULY DISEASES

Apoplexy—same as sudden death in June hints. Old stock going light—results of last fall's cured (?) cases of colds and roup.

Summer colds and snuffles among growing chickens are the results of too hot sleeping quarters.

Be sure their feet rest on the ground, and not on board floors, and that they are never over warm.

About all they need is wire to protect them from the skunks, etc.

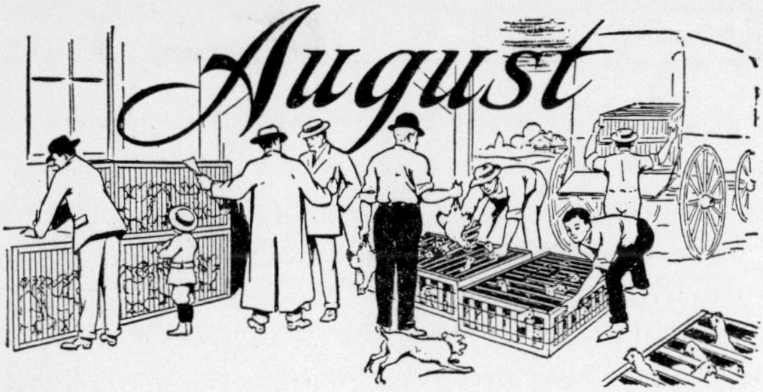

STARTING IN AUGUST

STARTING in August for table eggs, we should not recommend purchasing matured birds as it is just in the middle of the moulting period, and moving them about would result in stopping their laying altogether. Better get the house ready and purchase some early hatched pullets that will get to laying in September or October.

For breeding stock, this month is a good time to pick up some yearlings of some good reliable breed that suits you. They will make ideal stock for next season's use, begin laying in November or December, just in time for broilers and early winter work.

GENERAL SUGGESTIONS

When the poultrymen all find out that the first year of a layer's life is the most profitable, they will begin to market their old hens as fast as they start moulting. They should push them hard the first year, then buy or raise pullets to take their place. Early moulters are frequently slow moulters, taking eight to ten weeks for the process, while the later moulters will get through in half the time. Send them along to market as

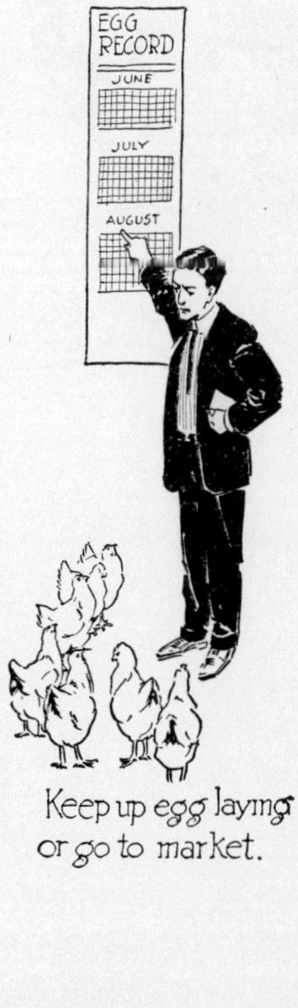

Keep up egg laying or go to market.

soon as they show signs of moulting and get pullets to fill their place. All the old surplus stock should now be marketed.

It is somebody's fault if the little summer chicks are dying.

The tender little fellows cannot withstand heat and lice combined. Protect them from the sun and get after the lice.

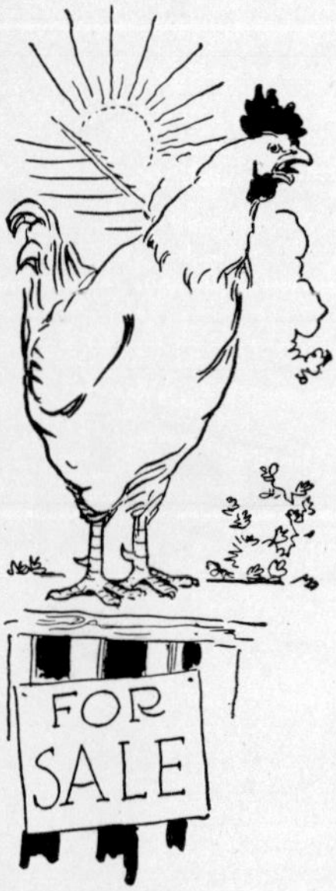

The old rooster crows well, but he is a tyrant. Either sell him or get him away from the laying hens some other way. He pesters them so that they cannot do their best.

Hot, dry weather, and larger chicks in with them, make it a hard condition for the later broods to catch up with the early ones, and a good many times it causes the owner to say, "Late chickens are no good anyway."

Late chickens are all right and as good money makers as the early ones, if properly cared for, but they must have radically different treatment when hatched in hot weather.

With the early birds we must take care to keep the pens dry, and their feet *off* the ground when being brooded. Late chicks must be kept cool, and after a few weeks old we must be careful to keep their feet *on* the ground when being brooded.

See that the growing stock has plenty of room to expand. Be sure that every chicken you own has plenty of elbow room to grow in and see that he is never overheated after nightfall. This is a bad month for crowded quarters. Often the seeds of next winter's crop of roup are sown in this month, simply by keeping the youngsters crowded into quarters about the right size for one-fourth the number. Results: the chickens are too hot at night and take cold by getting out on a chilly morning in September and waiting around for the sun to warm them up.

August is a good money making month. Prices of poultry are at good paying figures; eggs bring better returns and chickens hatched this month make splendid roasters during February and March. August hatched pullets will be found rather more profitable if turned for market than kept as layers.*

Shade, green stuff and plenty of water are all very essential for August chickens of all ages and sizes. Keep the different sizes by themselves.

There is no crop we know of that will produce such returns in green feed for poultry as Dwarf Essex Rape. Sow at any season of the year, wet or dry, hot or cold. Frost does not hurt it, and it will make a satisfactory growth anywhere, but with good rich soil and plenty of room the plants will soon rival cabbages in size, and remind one of loose-headed cabbages. Ask your seedsman for the seed.

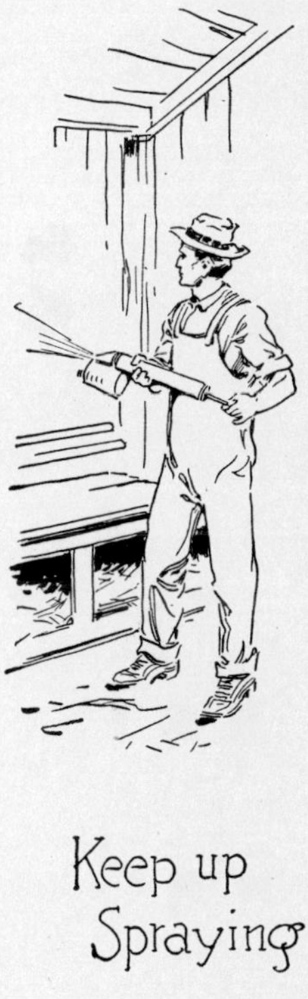

Keep up Spraying

Tell your neighbors of the results you obtain from good feeds and supplies. It will help them, and in helping them you help yourself, for if your neighborhood has the reputation of producing top-notch quality you will get better prices for your stock.

---

* A "layer" is a hen or pullet devoted to market eggs, not destined to be used in the breeding pen.

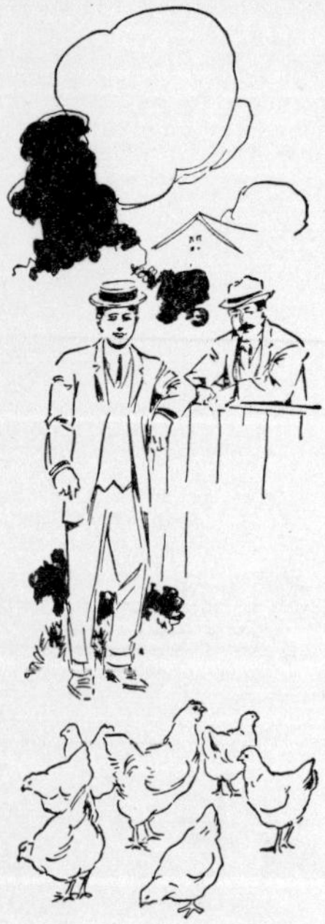

Tell your neighbor about your success

Begin to market the old hens as they stop laying. Be sure that they are good and fat, as per suggestions in July.

This is a bad month for mites.

Use a sprayer for applying liquid lice killer and some disinfectant to the various houses and runs. A good sprayer makes thorough, quick and easy work. Pay special attention to spraying the nest boxes and the perches.

AUGUST DISEASES

Whenever you can do so, separate your chickens into smaller flocks, and if you want any particular lot to develop especially quick, divide them once more.

The smaller the number together, the less trouble, and the most results.

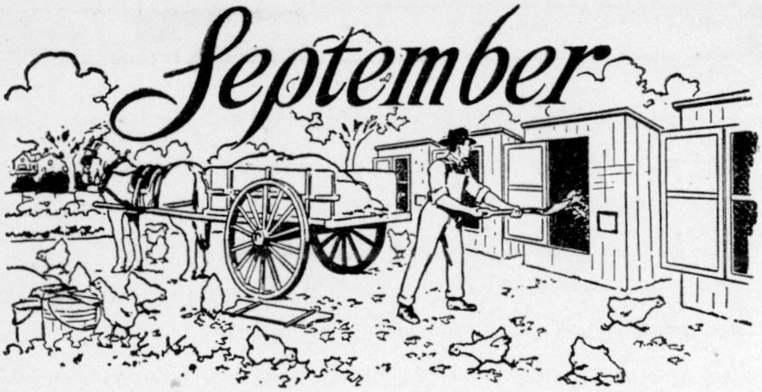

STARTING IN SEPTEMBER

STARTING in September, buy pullets for family eggs, and yearling hens for the best breeding stock for another season. Buy house and other appliances as in other months, but support the house on posts and get sand or gravel in early before the fall rains wet it. House your birds that are intended only for laying, but let the breeding stock have all the range outside the house that you can provide.

Hatch a few broods of chicks this month. They will lay in March and keep at it until Fall. Winter them in a house by themselves, with plenty of food by them at all times. Sell the cockerels in February.

GENERAL SUGGESTIONS

Get the early March-hatched pullets that you plan to use for layers into winter quarters by the middle or last of this month.

There never will be too many good poultrymen; do not be afraid of that. Be one of the best.

It is not too late to get another litter out of the hens that have not moulted yet.

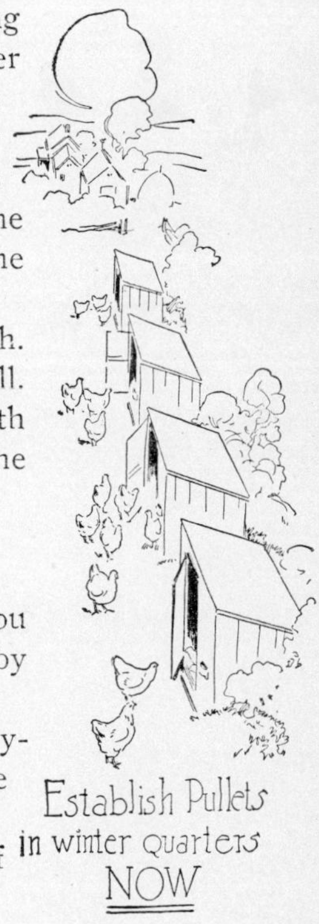

Pullets are worthy of your best attention. Get the early ones into winter quarters, and contented this month.

It checks them less to move them before they begin to lay.

Yard the cockerels by themselves; not only the market stock but the ones you have selected for breeders. They grow much better than when placed with the pullets or hens. If they begin to get scrappy, put in one of the old cocks with them. He will maintain order, and is tickled with "his job."

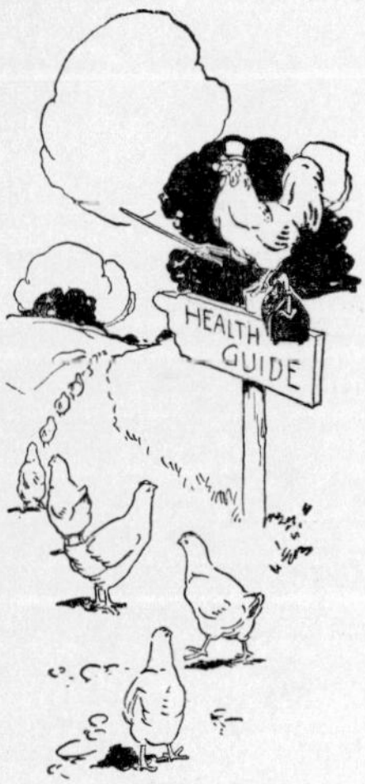

Keep them Healthy

This is the time the wet mash hen goes to pieces, so to speak. While her dry fed sister is laying right along, she takes a complete vacation, loafs around, neither an ornament nor help, demonstrating the truth of our claim of healthier flocks by this system of feeding. We repeat last month's warning; keep the chickens cool nights, do not let them pile up or sweat, see them personally at least once a week, and provide plenty of room. Get them out of the trees as soon as the nights get frosty; put them in winter quarters, but keep the house cool.

Keep working off the old hens, watch your flock of growing youngsters. If you find a number that lag behind the others, put them by themselves and see that they have a little better chance.

Have your houses all cleaned out, and put in about six inches of clean sand or loam.

Keep the hens happy and healthy. Use liquid lice killer, and some good disinfectant.

Hens with scaly legs are undesirable mothers.

Get the capons to market, for prices are now on the downward scale, and it does not pay to hold them once they are in condition.

March pullets should be laying this month.

Keep track of the different lots of cockerels, and your different breedings by a system of banding the birds.

We do not advocate warm poultry buildings, but we do insist that they must be dry and free from draught.

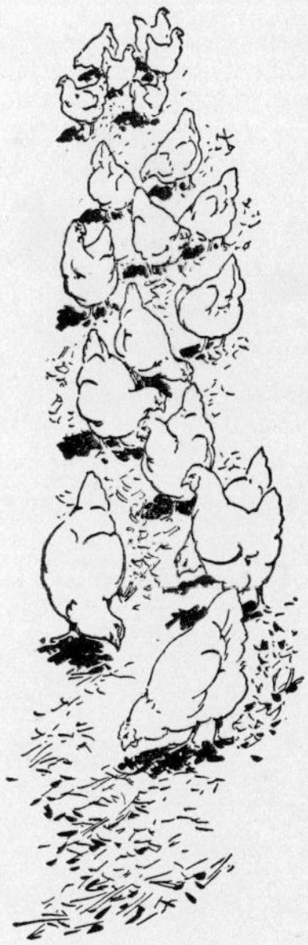

Now the July pullets of last year will give a nice yield of eggs at prices that pay handsomely. If for table eggs let the birds stay in the house all summer, in fact after they go into winter quarters never let them out of the house again, and you will get a larger egg yield.

Begin to get things pulled together for winter; it is some ways off but it will soon be here.

Eggs getting scarce and higher.

September-hatched chickens should be brooded in small brooders and coops.

Prepare the hens now for fall and winter laying. Prepare the pullets also.

Each brood of chickens from one year's end to another should have a new spot of land to grow on, but this is particularly true of late or hot-weather hatches. Be sure all roofs over your plant are tight; if not, make them so. Change the sand or gravel before the fall rains, and whitewash or disinfect all winter quarters.

Most buyers make the mistake of not providing enough space for the youngsters after they hatch.

Get the regular fall cleaning done and by the latter part of the month have everything ready for a quick shift if there is need.

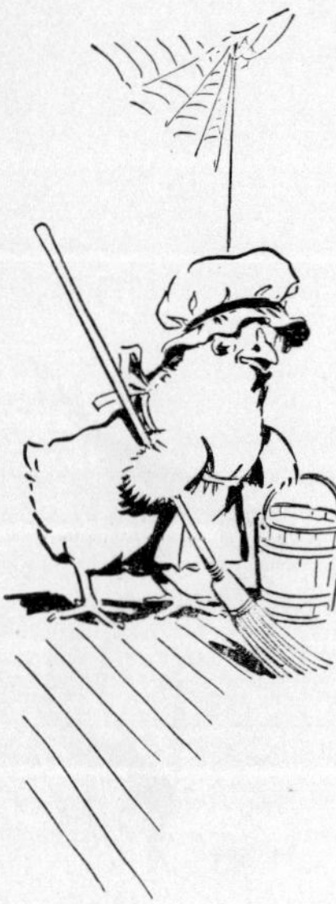

More birds start in the wrong direction and toward a winter sickness in September than in any other month.

Keep up a spraying.

Feed every atom they will eat.

SEPTEMBER DISEASES

The way to cure colds and roup is to prevent them. See that your stock is always cool at night with plenty of roosting room, and watch them carefully when you move them—that they don't get overheated in bags or boxes.

"Going-Light" is a diseased condition that is hard to cure, caused by too much poor quality meat supply. The axe is about the best remedy.

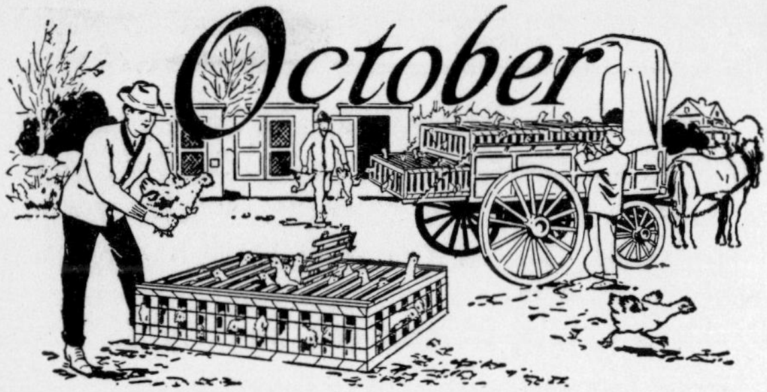

STARTING IN OCTOBER.

Starting in October, get your house in order as soon as you can. Then buy well matured pullets to provide table eggs, and the mixed varieties will do just as well as the more expensive, full-blooded breeds. For breeding stock, purchase only full blooded, either yearlings or well matured pullets will be satisfactory. Give breeding stock plenty of exercise out of doors daily. Layers should be kept closed in.

GENERAL SUGGESTIONS

This is the right month to have your winter layers start in. If they begin much earlier than this they are not as good layers as a rule, and sometimes get broody and moult.

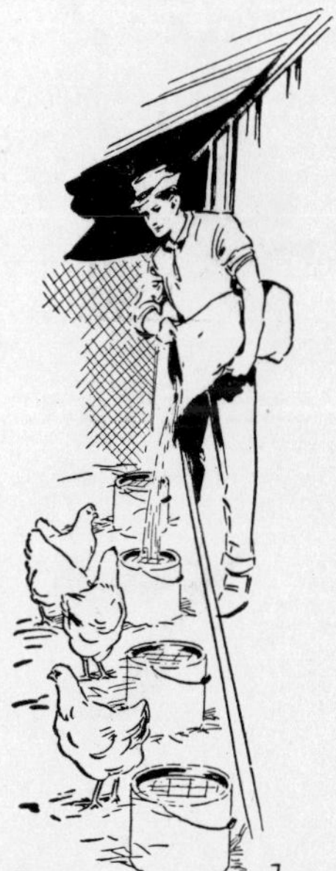

Eggs steadily increasing in price.

Divide the pullets into small flocks, being careful to keep each size and age and color by itself, for best results—unless mixed colors have been raised together. The smaller the flock, the faster they will develop.

Eggs steadily advancing in price and giving good profits, in fact as good as during the cold winter season.

Live poultry dealers in all the large cities take care of all the odds and ends. Send them the old hens, old cocks, chickens, surplus pullets, in fact, everything you wish to turn into cash. Ship them alive.

Keep only what you can properly feed and care for—especially feed.

Use plenty of good litter, the birds need exercise to keep in the condition that means profitable poultry.

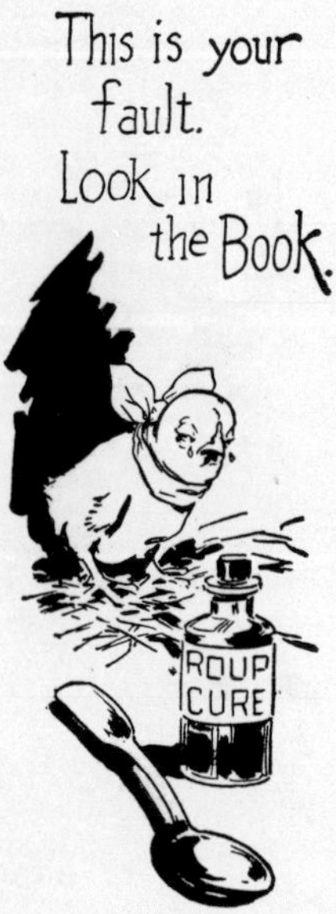
This is your fault. Look in the Book.
ROUP CURE

Many bad cases of roup are started this month by allowing the chicks to lie around under the bushes in damp places. Better yard any that show a tendency to act this way, feed liberally, and use Roup Cure in drinking water.

Keep the late chicks in the coops these frosty mornings.

Feed them early before letting out.

If breeding from pullets, mate with large, healthy, 2-yr. old cocks. There is no better mating than this.

Some chickens grow one end at a time and during their early days are sometimes all legs, while later they mature into quite well proportioned stock; then again some of them have the appearance of standing still and making little progress for a month or more, when they shoot ahead again. All these should be weeded out, and a quick-growing, hearty-eating bird that was well proportioned at four or five pounds chosen.

Select your next season's breeders now, and choose the ones that have made the most rapid growth as youngsters, i. e., the ones that have reached the four to five pounds' weight in the least number of days.

This does not mean the undersized, small, precocious chap that gets "cocky" when very young. These are the very ones that you should avoid, for they will run the size of your stock down very rapidly if bred from. Choose rather the male bird that does not discover that he is a male until six or seven months of age. He has been busy putting bone and muscle together and he will make the right kind of chickens that do not "go hard" young.

In the latitude of New England poultry should be in their winter quarters this month and everything snug and in shape for the cold winter which is now liable to come at any time.

The secret of success is hard feeding and cleanliness. Keep up their appetites and keep down the vermin.

Gather the leaves for litter.

The farmer will have some cabbage that did not head up very well. It is just what you want. Spread it on the north side of the house and cover with about a foot of hay and leaves.

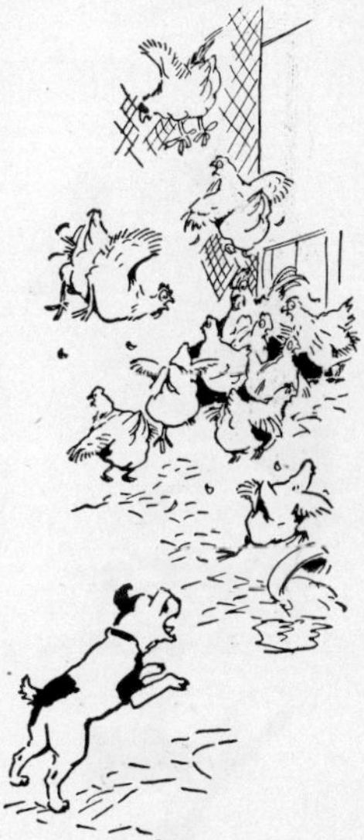

Never allow a scare.

Never allow anyone or anything to scare the chicks or fowl.

If you are not getting a satisfactory egg yield see if you are housing and feeding your stock right. Be sure all the chickens are out of the trees before the cold rains start in, and when changing birds from the trees into the houses, see that the houses are as cold as they can be kept during the nights without having draughts striking the birds on the roosts.

All your birds should be in winter quarters this month. The earlier March hatches should have been under cover last month and should now be laying quite steadily. It is always better to house them a month or six weeks before they begin to lay, for fall laying is against Nature's law and on the slightest provocation she steps in and puts an end to the unnatural production and it is hard work to regain the ground lost.

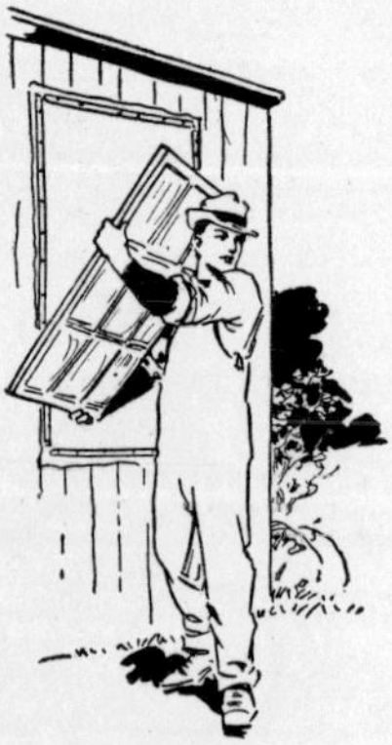

Windows out substitute waterproof sheeting.

OCTOBER DISEASES

The one worst feature of the long houses is the tendency to draughts, and the likelihood of canker and other contagious troubles working from one pen to another. We prefer isolated flocks for money making every day in the year.

When you move the pullets into winter quarters, be sure that they are cool at night. Take out the windows, but see that they are not in a draught on the roosts.

November

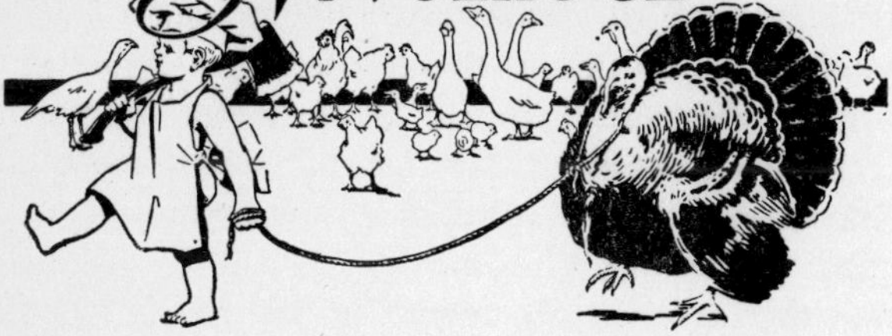

STARTING IN NOVEMBER

STARTING this month, we find eggs at the extreme high figures of the year, and pullets or yearlings are very slow in commencing to lay. The night constitutes almost two-thirds of the twenty-four hours and it is hard for the birds to eat enough in the brief day to make up for the long nights and lay eggs at the same time.

Get your house in position as quickly as possible.

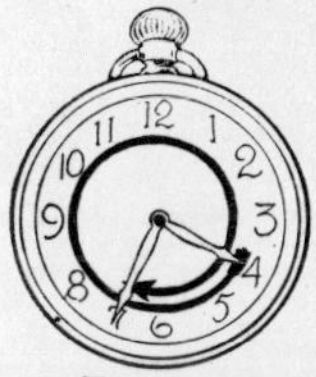

15 FEEDING HOURS IN SUMMER AGAINST

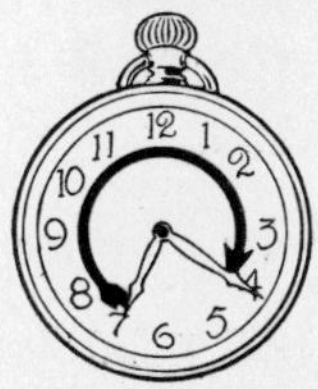

9 FEEDING HOURS IN WINTER

Be sure to have plenty of litter, so that your birds' feet never get on the cold ground; but still don't overdo it, for they will not scratch as well if litter is too deep. Just right is when they scratch down to the gravel every day.

Buy your breeding cockerels this month, and get the first selection, and also be ready to get out the early broilers.

GENERAL SUGGESTIONS

Be sure every old hen is marketed before this month is out unless you want them for breeders another season, and fill up with pullets that pay better.

Years ago, and not so many at that, we all

got up early, a lot before daylight, and started boiling water under the big kettle. Then we lugged the mash around to each pen, and we put down just what they would eat up clean in five minutes. We had shutters for the windows, roosting closets, every crack and crevice sealed up tight, warmed the water and the grain.

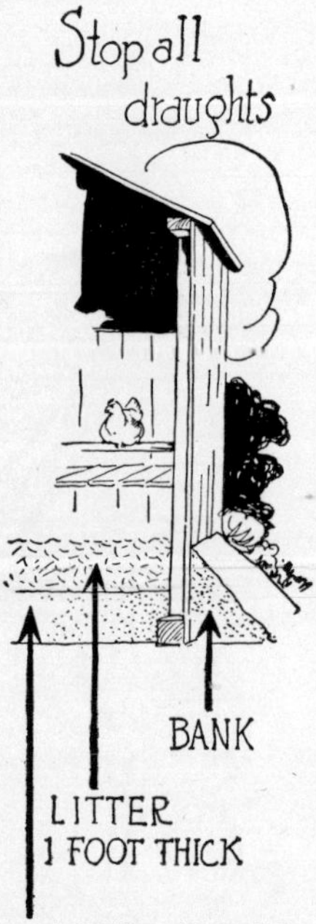

Think of the steps we took, and then we didn't get half as many eggs as we do today with Egg Feed, open front houses, and cold water, Egg Feed fed once a week, and the hens are a lot healthier, our health is better, too, and our profits are more than double.

November is a month of long nights and short days; while during the summer months the birds are on the roosts eight hours or less and are busy eating the other sixteen, now the reverse is the rule and they should not be kept waiting a minute for the owner or attendant to feed them. The dry ground feed is always there, and as soon as it is light enough they can begin filling up, and naturally they are at it from morning until night. No chance for a feast, then a famine, as under the old system. This is why results are so much more certain with this method.

Thousands of women are engaged in poultry keeping, finding it a sure and profitable method of making money, and city markets for live poultry remove all the disagreeable features of killing and marketing the birds.

See that your house is banked up around the bottom so as to avoid draughts.

One of the best helps toward keeping the quarters dry in winter, at a nominal cost, is to have the floor well littered to the depth of from three to six inches with dirt, cut straw, hay or leaves. This protects against loss of heat and prevents cold currents from below, and may also be used in which to scatter the grain to keep the fowls active.

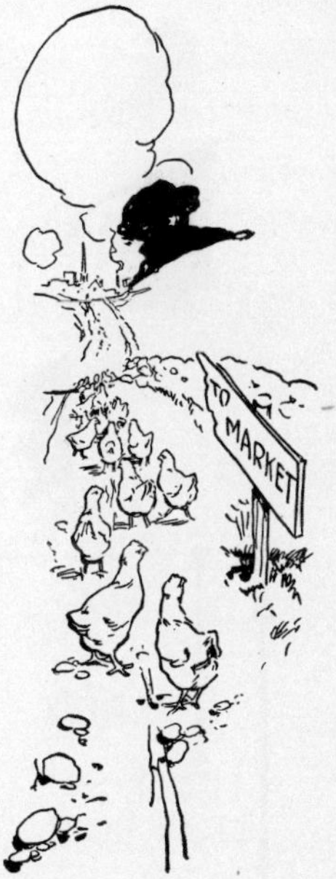

You should be getting a good supply of eggs from March and April pullets and the May-hatches should be starting in. Keep the different ages by themselves so that the younger ones are not "bossed" around. Kept separated they will mature much faster.

Push everything to market early this month, as the late holiday markets are seldom satisfactory, except for very large choice eight to nine-pound fancy capons. These it might pay to hold, but really they should have gone to market two months ago when prices were better. July and August chickens should be pretty well feathered out and able to care for themselves if properly housed.

Eggs bring long prices this month and poultry is at the low point for the year.

November is, on the whole, a bad month to market fowl and chickens. Turkeys have the right of way, and so many unposted producers rush in fowl and chickens that the market is usually glutted and prices run low.

The more vigorous the male, the larger the percentage of good pullets from the mating.

The poultry will stand almost any degree of

cold, but draughts mean sure trouble. If there is any sign of a cold, use some roup cure.

Keep the hoppers full. The hens are keeping union hours now. They say the way to a man's heart is through his stomach. You must jolly the hen the same way.

Better gather your eggs for hatching several times a day; during this kind of weather eggs quickly chill.

Treat the pullets the best you know how and your reward will be sure and ample.

Give your birds plenty of air, with the south side open day and night.

It is not always necessary to supply grit, but as it is so cheap, you cannot afford to take chances. The hens need it for best results.

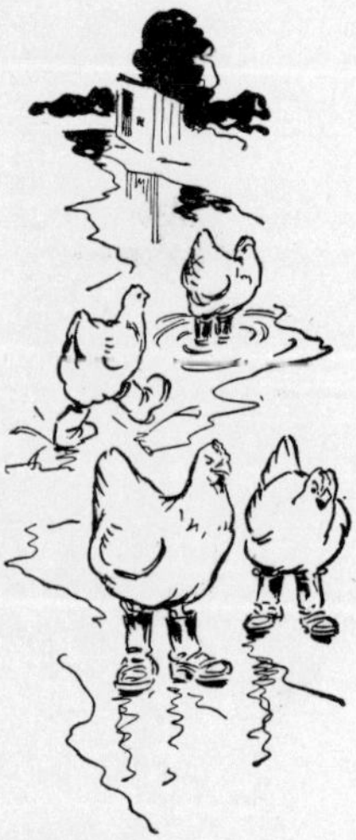

Dry feet — plenty of Eggs

NOVEMBER DISEASES

Getting out on the cold ground, walking around in the snow and slush, damp litter, all stop your birds from laying. Don't try to keep your birds warm but keep them dry at whatever cost. Keep them scratching.

The circulation of the blood is very active through the hen's foot, and she cannot devote her feed to making eggs if it takes too much of it to keep her feet warm.

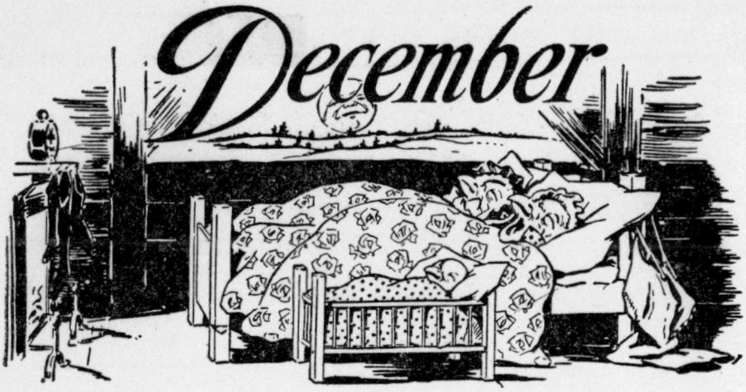

STARTING IN DECEMBER

Starting in December is much like starting in January and the same rules as November apply. Depend upon early hatched pullets to get eggs this month. Keep the birds dry. Get strong, fertile eggs from yearling hens. Don't put over eight females with a male at this season of the year.

Get them all out of doors every day and the eggs will hatch much better. Dig off the snow in front of the coop, making a space equal in size to the size of the pen. Feed them Scratch Feed outside in some litter so they will scratch in the open air for it. This means some extra work, but fertile eggs in winter are worthy of a good deal of extra labor.

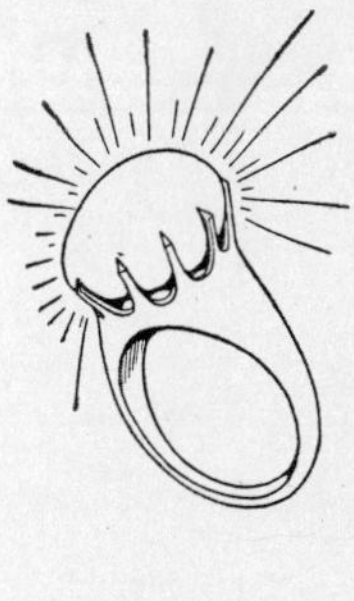

GENERAL SUGGESTIONS

Cut out the leaks, not only in the coop, but in your business. If you have a lot of old hens that do not look like laying right away, market them.

This is the month when "eggs is eggs."

If you have a lot of cockerels that are not big enough for breeders, or any old cocks that you are not going to use, market them.

Get your birds into small flocks. Get them settled down for the winter. Get late hatched pullets in place of two-year-old hens. They will pay better.

Don't let your market egg layers out of doors under any condition during the winter months, and keep their pens well littered. There is a wonderful lot of blood circulating through their feet, and they won't lay if they stand around in mud and snow all day.

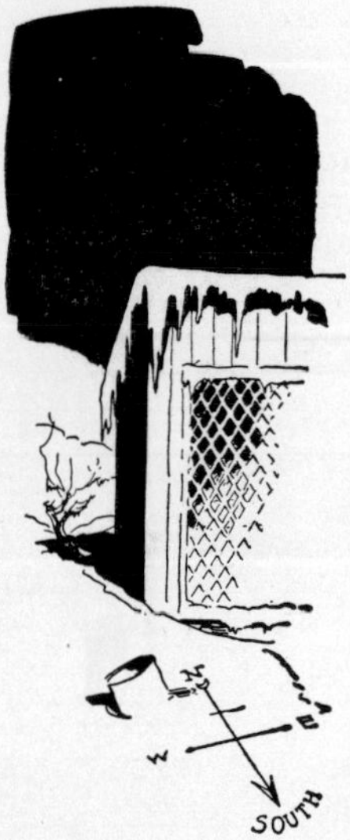

Whether you believe it or not, this is allright.

Keep in airy houses with liberal sized openings in the south side which are never closed night or day.

In selecting breeders for the broiler or roaster that is to be hatched next month, choose the male as per suggestions in October, and select females that are of good size, hardy, vigorous breeders, birds that from the shell up have never known what it was to lose a feed. We strongly favor the large American varieties for all purposes, for they lay as well and make much better poultry than the smaller breeds. Select hens, yearlings, that are well through the moulting and about ready to lay, or pullets that have been well matured before starting to lay, thus insuring good sized eggs; mate not over six or eight females with a male that has been kept away from all females until this time, and the chances are you will get eggs that will hatch those strong, rugged chickens that will live through tornado, earthquakes and blizzards.

December and January-hatched chickens mature in June, bringing highest prices of the year.

Keep charcoal in front of your poultry all the time.

Vigor is only another way of spelling health. If your breeders are healthy, strong birds, and your house is open so that they practically roost and live in the open air twenty-four hours a day, and if you feed as we direct, the chickens will be vigorous and healthy, and you will raise every one you put in small heatless brooders.

Have you purchased your stock of breeding cockerels? It's a good time now before the stock gets culled over.

Keep the hens busy. Dry leaves make the best kind of litter.

It is nice to have the house whitewashed so that it will not be so dark on stormy days.

Sort over your pullets and if you have more than you can take care of properly, send the surplus to market.

Keep an egg record. Try to have an intelligent idea of what your poultry costs you and what it returns.

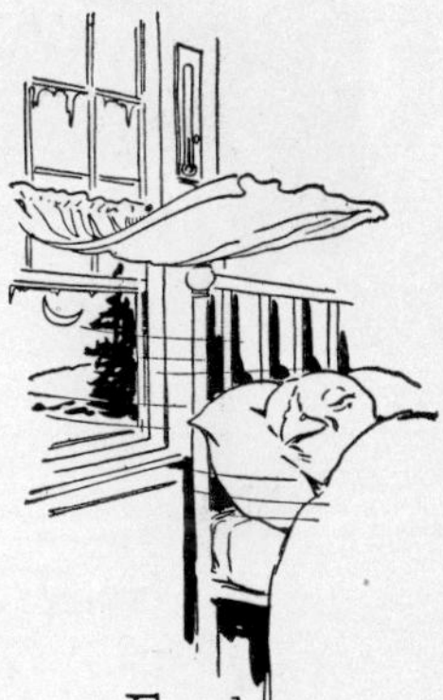

Fresh air for Poultry too.

See that you have plenty of eggs and that the poultry is all marketed or is growing along to maturity for the better prices of another season.

This is the month of highest prices for eggs and bottom prices for poultry.

It is a good idea to use some roup cure in the drinking water. "Prevention is better than cure."

See that your birds are eating every minute of the time from leaving the roosts until they get back on them, for they now spend nearly

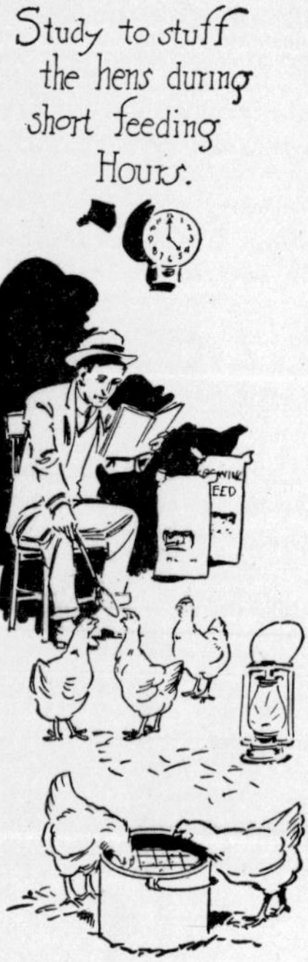

two-thirds of their time on the perches and must eat continuously to get enough to lay all the eggs you expect.

Accept our hearty wishes for a happy New Year.

DECEMBER DISEASES

In December practically the only disease to guard against is roup, and this is really the only one in the business to fear—and fear this we must, as it is the worst of them all; in fact is worse than all the others combined, and at that it is a disease resulting from carelessness or ignorance.

Give the birds good air to breathe at all times, treat them as though they were hardy and strong from the time they are hatched, and they will be strong and free from disease.

Baby them, pamper them, raise them in heated buildings, keep them in tight houses—and you will have continuous trouble.

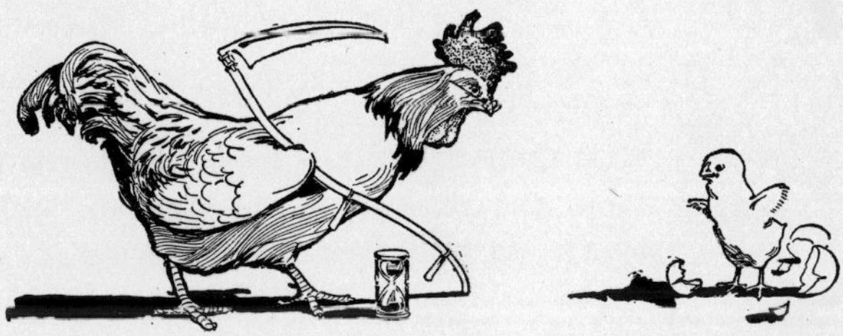

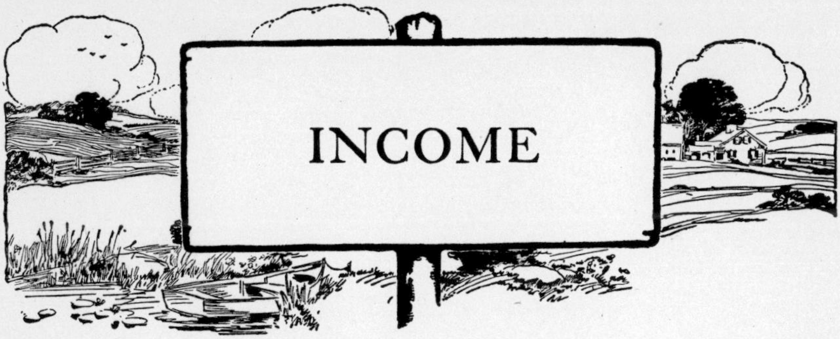

INCOME

VITALITY is largely inherited, and without vitality our work and pains are thrown away. If we do not have good, strong parent stock the chickens will be weak, puny things that are worse than useless. Experienced poultrymen will testify that such stock is of no value; in fact, is a curse to anyone, their care nothing but a continual worry, and their survival only a deferred disappointment. Better pay double the price for good, strong, robust stock than to have the other kind given to you.

Assuming that you have the kind of stock described above, and that the chickens are hatched, we will try to outline a simple system of care and management that will bring them to laying in good season.

Now, to get early fall and winter eggs, or in fact to get any kind of success with poultry, we must study nature and her methods.

You have all noted that Red-root or Pigweeds that come up in a vacant lot late in September or October have a different habit of growth than when beginning to grow in the early spring. In the spring the habits of the

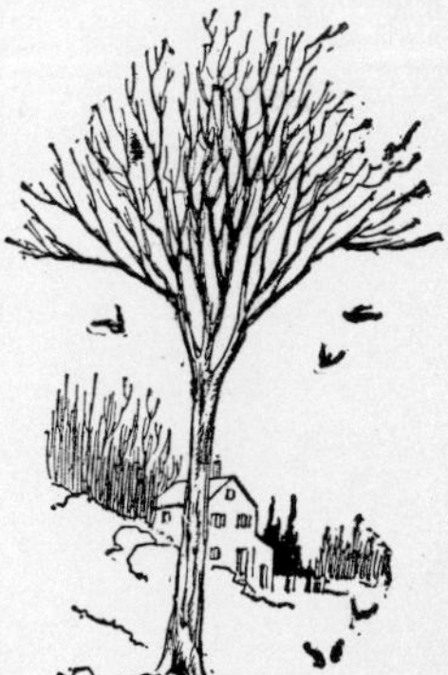

You never see a Robin build a nest during the fall months.

plant are apparently on the broad gauge plan. The branching stalks and main stem are wide and thick, intended to grow to large size before bearing seed, and if left unhampered to grow as started on rich soil, the plant will reach a height of 5 or 6 ft. before any blossom buds appear. Now the same seed in the same soil sprouting in October will grow with another plan of life altogether. Instead of the thick stem and branching habit it shoots up a small dwarf habit stem less than 6 inches in height before blossom buds appear. This is simply nature's recognition of the fact that the growing season is past, that the harvest time is near, and whatever seed is borne must be produced in haste. The plant's form is shaped with this end in view, and is brought to bearing in its limited time and on a dwarfed frame.

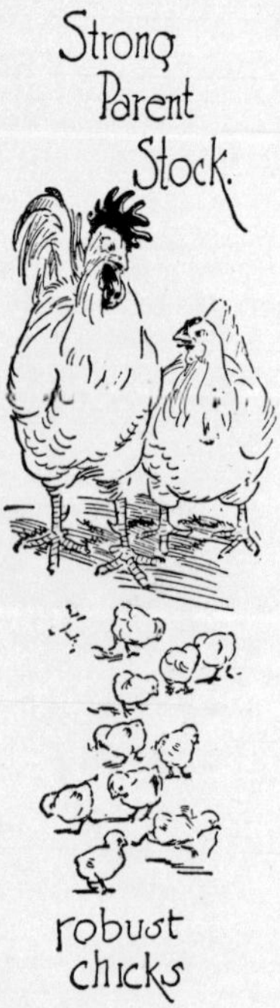

Now, the springtime is nature's season of breeding. Among practically all the wild animals the young are produced during the spring months. It matters very little when your pullets are hatched, they will lay in February, March and April anyway. If these chickens are hatched in May, June or July and improperly fed or half starved, allowed to shift for themselves, they will come to laying during these months. The same is true of August, September or October-hatched pullets. They too will lay in February, March and April, but they will not be so well developed. Their bodies will be small, and their eggs will be undersized. So too, will pullets hatched in January and February get to laying in May or June. Nature, recognizing the Spring as the breeding or producing season, hurries these birds, hatched, according to her calendar, late on the last growing period, and sets them to laying, very small eggs to be sure, but eggs, and eggs that will hatch. Of course the pullets are small, and never make the frames they would have grown had they been hatched at the proper season.

This is simply to show that nature has a period of seed time, of growth, and another of harvest or maturity. Now, she times that period of growth with all her children when the feed is most plentiful. You never see the robin or bluebird, the deer or moose building nests or bearing young at any other time than during the early spring or summer when the feed is most abundant, giving the young ample time and feed for maturing before the winter season.

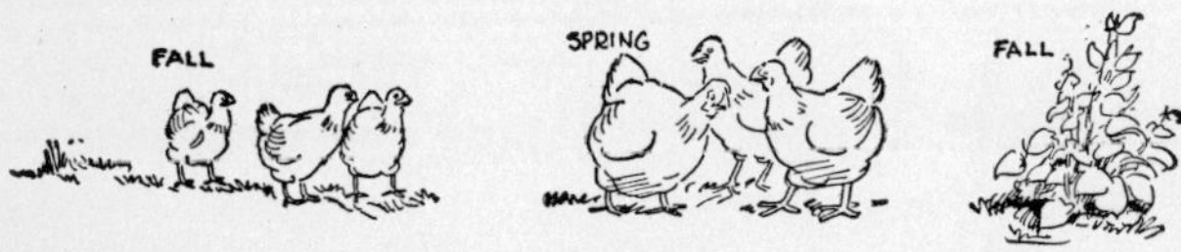

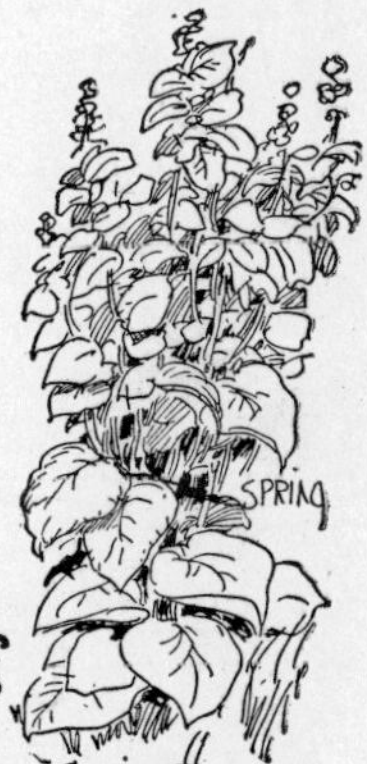

Spring growth versus Fall growth

Now, man in his manipulation of nature's laws, as regards the hen, by creating an abnormal appetite and laying habit, has a bird that under some conditions breeds or produces eggs in the off season or fall and winter months. Left to herself to pick her own living the hen would only lay during the spring and summer months, and we are sure that those eggs would hatch much better than those produced by our perpetual machine that is laying five to ten times as many eggs as Nature intended her to.

The burning question is, why don't we get as many eggs during the fall and winter season as during the spring and summer? Really, is not the question, WHY DO WE GET ANY EGGS DURING THE FALL AND WINTER?

If we stop to consider the effects of years of breeding of our domestic animals we will find that the improvements have been along the line of increased capacity for food, resulting in increased productiveness. In the milch cow the development of her appetite and productiveness has probably increased her size 200 per cent. to 400 per cent., and her milk yield in the full year from 200 per cent. to 800 per cent. over cattle in a state of nature.

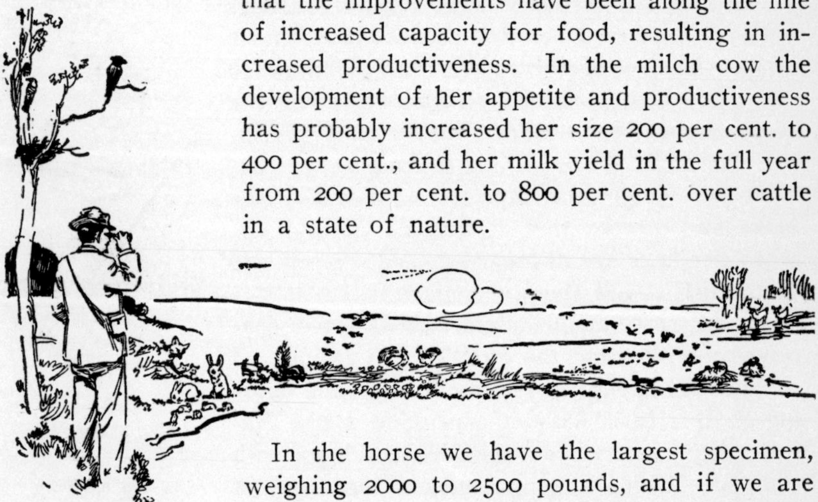

We must study nature

In the horse we have the largest specimen, weighing 2000 to 2500 pounds, and if we are to believe the naturalist these have been developed from animals weighing less than the little donkeys our children played with. Compare the old razor-back hog with enormous weight of some of the show Berkshire or White Chesters of today, weighing from 1000 to 1500 pounds.

All these cases cited sift down to man's manipulation and increase in the capacity of the animal to assimilate more feed than its ancestors and put it to the uses sought.

Now, in poultry just as wonderful changes have been wrought. In our domestic hen in place of the jungle fowl laying one or two clutches of eggs, perhaps 25 or 30 eggs in the spring months, we are not satisfied unless we get from 150 to 200 and want them all when eggs are at the highest prices.

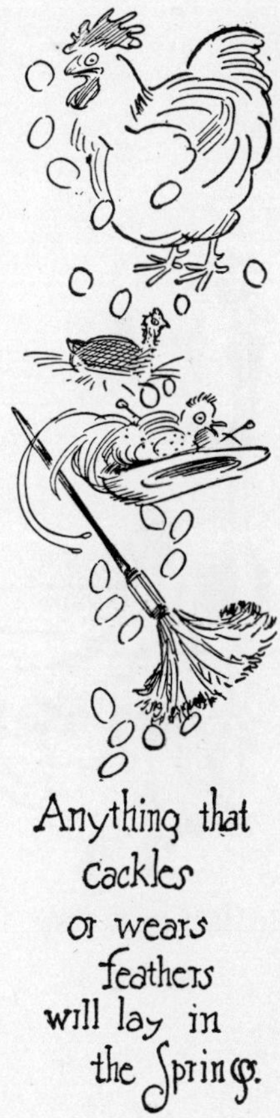
Anything that
cackles
or wears
feathers
will lay in
the Spring.

Mankind has certainly done wonderful things with our feathered pets but cannot stand nature on her head altogether. We must continue to court her favors and try to lead her along the road we wish her to follow, but we must remember that while she is willing as long as we consider her whims and caprices, occasionally she balks and wrecks our aspirations in mid air, when her laws are disregarded, and we come to earth with a dull thud.

In the past, amateur enthusiasts have conceived the idea that the birds laid in spring and summer because it was warm weather, and figuring on this basis without consulting Dame Nature, they constructed expensive buildings with elaborate heating systems, endeavoring to try to convince the birds that spring time had come, even if the sun did rise at seven o'clock and set at four. Their attempts have all failed for the very important reason that the birds were not adapted to live in stifled air and heated quarters, and that eggs are not dependent upon warmth. Colds, roup and kindred ailments put these plants out of business in short order.

To produce this five or ten-fold increase of egg yield over what nature intended, we must continue to crowd the right kind of feed into the birds in about the proportion we expect eggs.

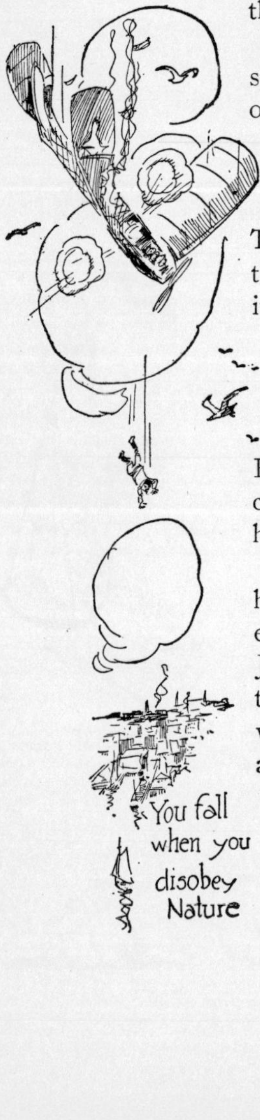

In the state of nature the birds hatched in the spring laid the next spring, or at about the age of ten months. Now we hear all kinds of protests if the pullets do not get to laying at five and six months of age, and in many cases where they have not been more than half fed at that. Taking ten months to develop in a mild climate they required very little feed and effort to secure it, especially as the birds were very much smaller than our birds of today. One of our American variety pullets should weigh from five to six pounds at six months of age. The jungle fowl weighed perhaps 2½ lbs. at ten months of age. How much more food must our well-bred bird consume to double this Jungle fowl's weight in half the time?

Supposing our American variety pullets are hatched in March or April how soon may we expect them to lay? Nature would start the Jungle fowl with the intention of bringing her to laying maturity at ten months of age, and with a productiveness of perhaps twelve eggs as her first litter, and a weight of 2 lbs. to make. She would require probably less than 25 per cent. food and ten months to get it in. It's a long, slow, growing period with a lighter production at the end of it, soon broken up with three weeks of incubation.

We expect Miss Plymouth Rock to start laying promptly at nine o'clock in the morning of the day she is five months of age, and continue one egg a day during the short winter days when she has about 7 hours on the floor of the pen and 17 hours on the roost, until the next spring or summer; not only that, but we wonder why the eggs don't hatch as many chicks as were put in the machine, and why the chicks die in the shell, and why they don't all live.

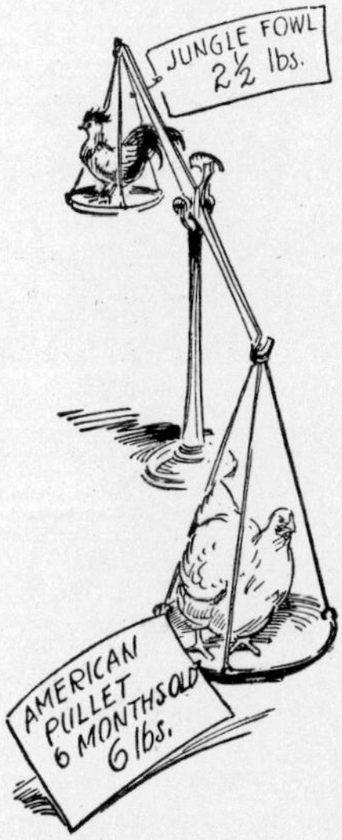

First of all, to bring Miss Plymouth Rock to laying at five to six months of age and have her up to the weight we wish, we must pour a constant stream of rich, nourishing food through her alimentary canal from the moment she is hatched. Every moment her digestive machinery is without material to build on is lost. If we start during infancy with scanty feeding, nature changes her plan from a wide-tailed big stocky bird to one of two-thirds or half the size, with a pinched and generally half-starved appearance.

We are very firm believers in the prenatal influence of full feeding. We think that to get heavy laying pullets, they must be well fed during their growing period else Nature thinks these birds are born to endure privation and short rations, and thus she dwarfs their future productiveness to suit the conditions under which they are developing.

If Miss Plymouth Rock is well started and pushed with the

right kind of food always within reach she will easily outgrow her ancestors, and having Nature always with her to prompt the development of her system for a period of plenty she will produce eggs of good size and frequency. But she must not be held back with unsuitable conditions or feed for a single moment from the shell up, and she must be kept in housing conditions that promote her steady addition to the natural hardiness inherited from her parents.

Hothouse conditions she cannot withstand, but given a suitable cold house with an abundance of fresh air, without draught, and plenty of food always within reach, she will lay more eggs than her ancestors, and go on as one of the links in the chain of the better producers we are seeking.

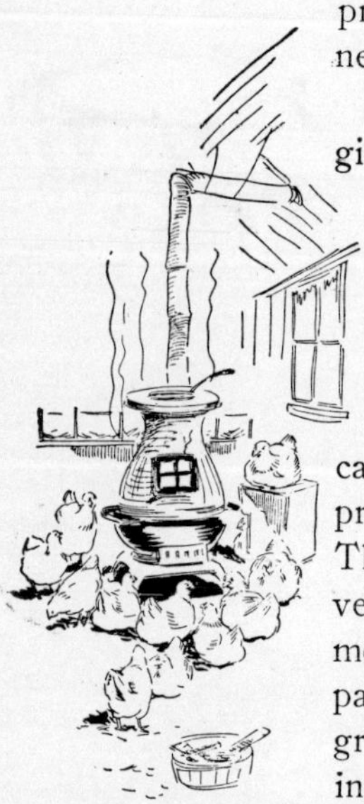

Nothing doing on the nests.

The birds are ravenous eaters, and what else can be expected if we consider what enormous producers they are when conditions suit them. They must have a large amount of feed to develop into this size and in the limited number of months we expect, and the feed must be rich, palatable and constantly before them. Whole grain will not produce the results we are looking for, since we have so increased the digestive capacity of the intestines, we have not yet greatly increased the efficiency of the gizzard, with the result that we must feed a large proportion of the feed in a finely ground state to give the intestines enough to do. Otherwise they are constantly waiting for the gizzard to send along some more material, and the result is lost ground, lessened growth and limited production.

Meat food is absolutely necessary. The growth and development we seek cannot and will not come from vegetable sources altogether. Animal protein we must have; and the only question remaining is in what form? We strongly advise the mixing of the meat food with the ground, whole grain, just as we have it in Growing Feed, years of study and experiment having demonstrated that this is the most palatable form, and productive of the maximum growth without any disturbance of the liver.

The birds in some sections get quite a little of their living from the grasshoppers and other bugs and worms, but be sure that in addition to this they always have some appetizing food constantly within reach so that the grasshoppers will be a little dessert and not the whole meal.

Be sure that a liberal percentage of the food is meat, from the hatch to the hatchet, and let it be meat of good quality.

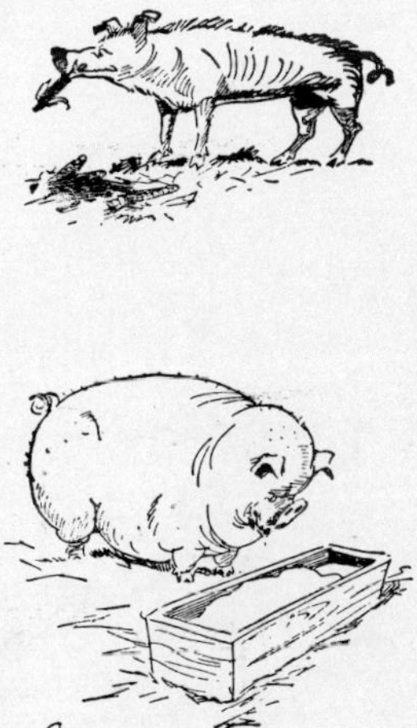

Compare "razor-backs" with Hogs of today

March or April-hatched pullets of the American varieties may or may not lay in September, October or November. If they have been well fed and properly cared for they will start laying during these months. On the other hand, if only half fed, allowed to find their own living, kept in small, ill ventilated quarters, crowded and stunted, or subjected to any one of the above handicaps, they will very likely hold back their eggs until the natural time for laying, February or March.

It is very easy to revert to the natural habit of spring and summer laying only. It requires good feed and care to overcome the natural tendency, and splendid returns come to those who master the problem.

Bringing the pullets along through the summer months in roomy, cool roosting coops, with plenty of green food and shade, and an abundance of rich, palatable food, always within easy access, the early fall months should see them rounding out into large, well-developed, wide-

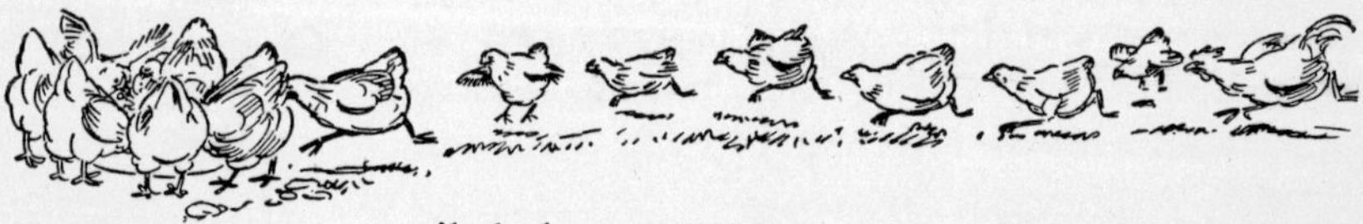

Hens are ravenous eaters.

tailed, henny-looking pullets that gain the size of their parents before beginning to drop their eggs. They have enjoyed full feeding during the natural growing period, and the fall finds them entirely matured and in the same state of development to which a scanty feeder would bring his birds in February or March.

We have taken advantage of Nature's teaching to grow the birds during the growing season, and she has rewarded us with a finished product in one-half the time she originally took to produce it. If we take the same pullet all ready to lay, transport her from one house to another, radically change the feed and care, our hopes may not materialize.

It is not the natural season for eggs, and too much abuse just as the birds are about to begin production will sometimes throw them back even so far as to wait until the spring season. It is best to get the pullets settled in their permanent winter quarters a month or more before they would lay, and after they have been placed together no change of the personnel of the pens permitted. Strangers introduced from time to time cause more or less scrapping and disturbance, and all go to interrupt egg production. During the unnatural season for eggs seemingly trivial matters and excuses cause the egg production to stop, whereas, during the flood tide of eggs in the spring season apparently one can go to almost any extreme with shifting, feeding, et cetera, without affecting the egg yield materially.

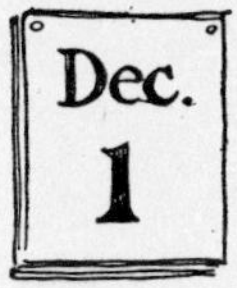

We may confidently expect eggs during the off season from early hatched pullets and from yearling hens that were early hatched the previous spring; having laid early during the preceding fall and winter they have been indifferent layers during the summer months, have moulted early and with proper feed and care are ready to begin their second season's work early.

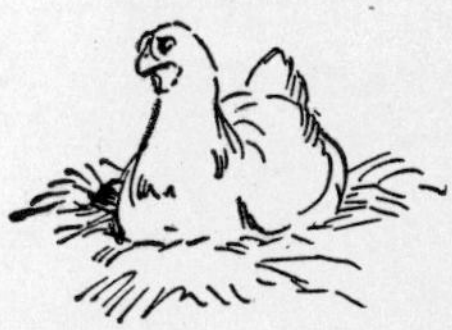

5 months to the day and minute they expect her to get on the nest and lay.

From the foregoing it would seem that only one class of pullets are desirable,—*the early hatched*. This, however, is not as we see it. We all like the early hatched, but we find that if our birds are all early hatched, within a reasonable space of time they will come to laying together, providing of course, that they all receive the same treatment. Again, they would all moult at the same period and we would be at a standstill for eggs.

We have seen the habits and natural tendencies with the early hatched pullet. Now let us consider another class of birds, heretofore regarded as of very little value,—the late hatched, or the June and July chickens. These have their work to do, and also do it just as well if we understand them.

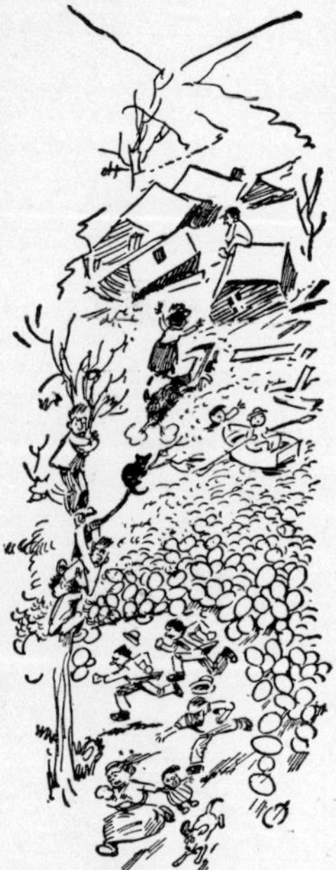

A flood-tide of eggs in the Spring

Carefully kept and well fed, they come to laying maturity in December, January and February. Beginning later, they go through the spring in better form, and when their early hatched sisters are moulting these late birds are still laying heavily, and as they have three months' time to make up, having begun three months later, they continue good, strong work right through August, September and October, stopping then for a short, quick moult, dropping the feathers almost all at once, and getting a new set very rapidly, whereas, the early hatched birds begin to drop their feathers in July or August and take three or four months for a very leisurely, ladylike change of clothing. To be sure they expose their bodies less, but the Salome dance ruling does not extend to the poultry yard, and results of the egg basket rather than beauty of bird are what we are seeking. It will be seen that the late hatched pullet fills her place and gives us eggs when they are quite scarce and hard to get. Prices are good and the eggs come with very little effort in feed and care.

Now if these pullets be purchased there is even more to be said in their favor. The early hatched are the kind that everybody is seeking, and the price is consequently bound to be high. These late ones are looked down upon, and not only bring a less price per pound, but as they are light in weight the total price is small indeed.

Put into the pens in October or November, weighing 2 to 3 pounds, they cost 40c. to 60c. each, while the early ones weighing 4 to 5 lbs. cost $1.00 to $1.25 each. Now when the time comes to go to market the early ones weigh about the same as when purchased, while the smaller ones have gained to about the size of the larger ones, and bring nearly, if not quite enough to purchase more small pullets to take their places.

The early ones must take quite a loss, as they are no more valuable as market poultry, cost quite a bit more per pound, and weighed heavier at the start. To be sure they got to laying earlier, but on the other hand they stopped earlier.

When the books are balanced at the end of the year it will be found that in many cases the late hatched birds have paid as much per head as the earlier ones. If these late hatched birds be wintered it will be found that they begin laying very nearly as soon as their medium early hatched sisters, and carry the same characteristics of late fall laying through the next season, although for this market egg business we favor the changing of the full stock each

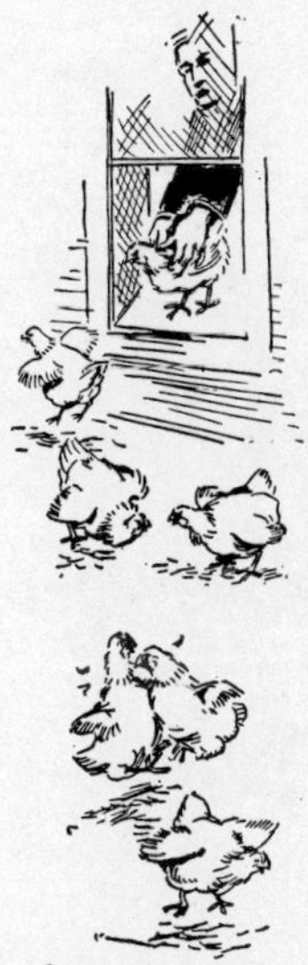

Disturbed Hens stop laying.

fall, either raising or purchasing an entire new lot.

We have tried to outline the natural tendency of the different classes of birds. Now, let us consider what we can do to increase the laying habit in the off season.

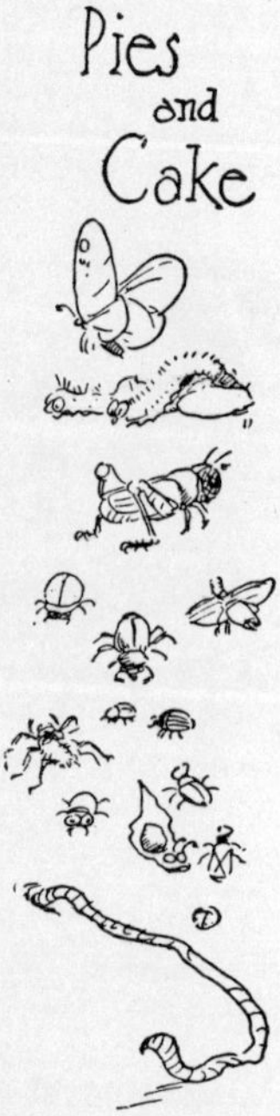

It will be acknowledged that almost everything from a feather duster to one of these new Easter bonnets will lay during the spring months. Anything that cackles and wears feathers and has half a chance to live will lay when Nature prompts her to do her best. For this reason we need take no credit upon ourselves for the large egg record during the spring months. The time for us to put out our best efforts is when Nature is urging her birds to "go slow" and take a rest.

We must push the early hatched pullets with liberal feeding of meat-laden food all through the growing period, then follow this with everything to whet her appetite and increase her productiveness while she is laying during the fall and winter. During the early spring she will lay anyway, for nature tells her to do so. But after the early spring is passed she is pretty nearly "all in" so far as eggs are concerned, and is either broody or loafing, laying very short litters between fits of broodiness or starting slow moults that will last for three or five months.

Now if in May we give her a change of diet,—for instance, shift from Egg Feed to a ration of Growing Feed with ten to fifteen per cent. of a good quality of meat scraps, the change of diet tickles her failing appetite and she eats ravenously of the new ration, gains flesh and lays a splendid lot of eggs during the following sixty days, when to our mind we have pretty well milked her out and she should go to market.

Now the late hatched birds as they are not allowed so much time during the growing period should be pushed harder, with, say a five or ten per cent. addition of scraps to the Growing Feed. They should be given yards and runs in which no birds have been kept for twelve months at least, and in smaller flocks than the earlier ones, not over 25 at most.

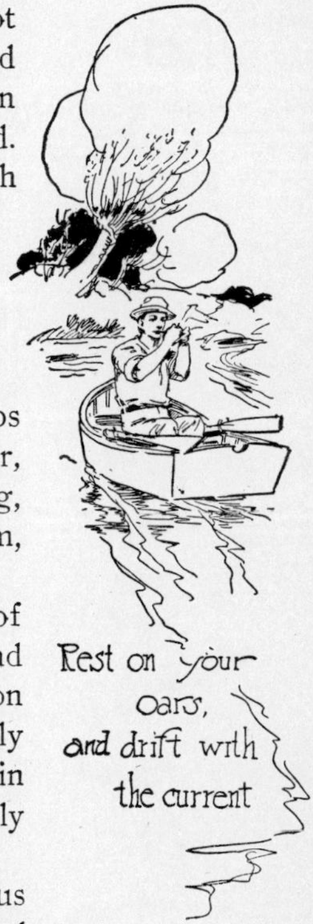

They have nature with them prompting the laying in February anyway, so we have only to encourage them with the extra ration of scraps to get them going a month or six weeks earlier, so we are seldom disappointed in their laying, usually getting eggs before we expect them, which is always pleasant.

During the spring months, like all the rest of poultrydom, they will lay under almost any kind of treatment and feed, so we had better rest on our oars and drift with the current until early summer, say about July, when we should begin the treatment previously outlined for the early hatched ones.

All our experience with poultry teaches us that the heavy feeders make the money, and any addition to the diet which will allow increased feeding with safety will more than correspondingly increase the profit.

OPPORTUNITY

THERE is much discussion of the steadily increasing cost of living, and with very good reason,—"it hits us where we live." For several years past the cost of all kinds of food stuffs has steadily increased, and this is especially true of beef, mutton and pork, which have advanced in price with alarming rapidity in the past few years. Nor is there any prospect of better conditions in these meat-foods, for the good and sufficient reason that a steadily increasing demand for food stuffs is met by a steadily diminishing supply of these products; to the inexorable law of supply and demand is due (in the main) the steady advance in prices.

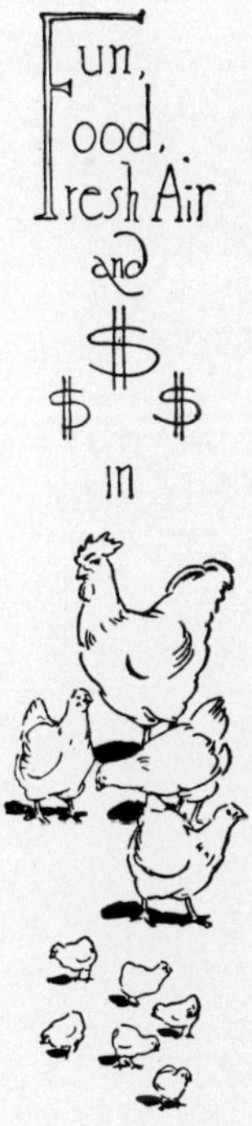

The population of the United States is increasing at a rate which means that each year there are a million more mouths to be fed than there were the year before. Over against this fact there has to be set the further fact of lessened production, due to the settling of the lands of the far west and south-west, and the turning of the great cattle and sheep ranges into small farms which are used for diversified farming, a factor which effects a change in the proportion of consumers to producers of food products, especially in the States east of the Mississippi River where the concentration of people in the cities and manufacturing towns is most marked. As it is apparent that it is the younger and more vigorous of the population who move to the towns and cities, so it becomes evident that not only the number but the efficiency of the producers is being diminished while an increased consumption has to be cared for.

Statistics furnished by the United States Department of Agriculture tell us that there were produced in 1910, 2,000,000 fewer beef cattle and 6,000,000 fewer hogs than were produced the year previous. The shrunken beef production is accounted for by the change in conditions in the west and southwest mentioned above; the lesser pork production is explained by the extremely high price, which induced the farmer to sell his young stock in place of making breeders of them.

This suburbanite thought he had no room for poultry keeping.

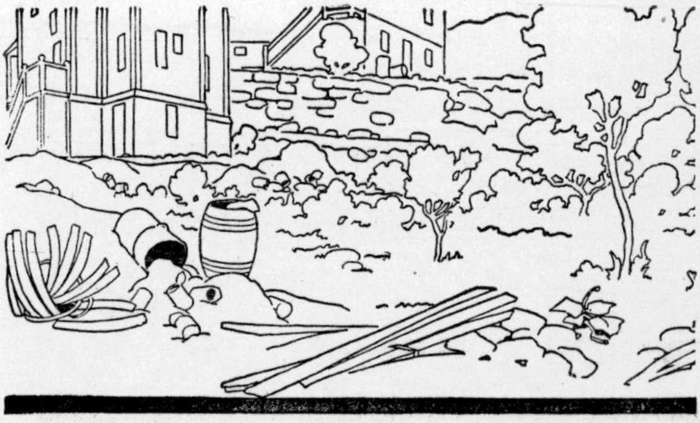

A natural outgrowth of this lessened food supply and increased demand is a turning to other sources of supply, foremost among which stand poultry-meat and eggs. That these articles of food are well appreciated is made evident by the fact that in the single state of Massachusetts there is consumed each year over $30,000,000 worth of them, and it is a very significant fact that only some five millions of dollars' worth of these products are grown within the state. That is to say, the people of the State of Massachusetts pay out each year over $25,000,000 for poultry-meat and eggs produced outside its limits.

In view of these facts it would seem wise for us to consider whether we cannot become producers of at least a portion of these foods, for our own households. Few of us realize the possibilities of a small flock of poultry in the back yard, and although we do realize the satisfaction there is in fresh-laid eggs for the breakfast table, we do not know how easily the eggs

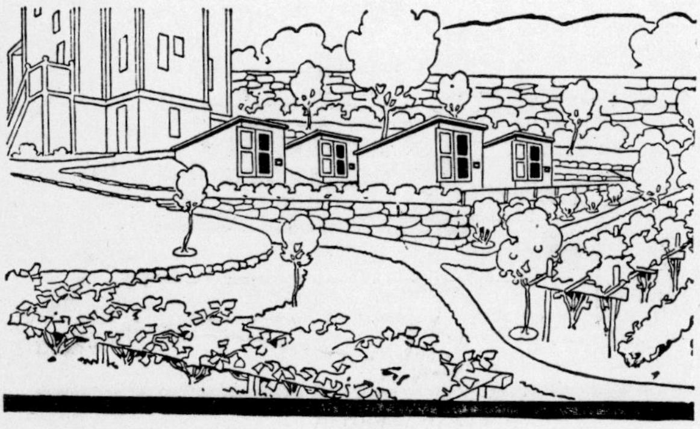

Same yard with four No-Yard houses and garden.

can be secured, nor how cheaply, at a cost of about a cent a piece for the food. The man who has a few square feet of room in the back yard may have the luxury of a constant supply of deliciously fresh eggs for the breakfast table and the family cooking at low cost, by simply taking advantage of the recent developments in methods of poultry keeping.

We all know the attractiveness, the delicious flavor of fresh-laid eggs, and how very far short of that attractive flavor are the cold-storage eggs which we receive, as "fresh" from the grocer or provision dealer. If it can be demonstrated that we can all have the genuine article, produced right in our own back yard at such small cost, surely we will hasten to add a small poultry house and flock of laying pullets to our possessions and become independent of the cold storage and semi-stale eggs previously experienced. Furthermore, we will eat decidedly more of them. Finding them eminently satisfactory, we turn to them again; they are "so

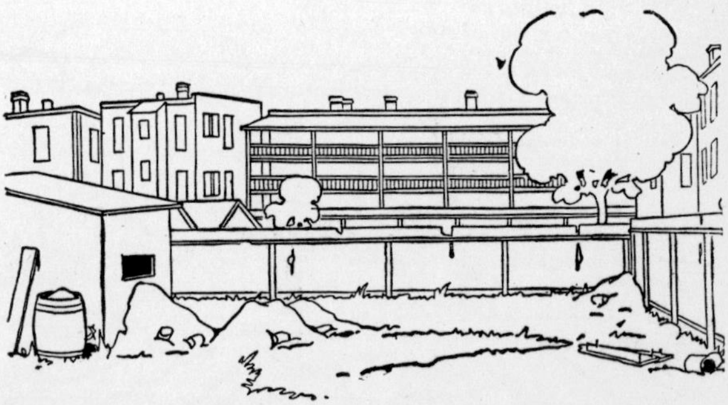

An unsightly back yard, producing nothing but regrets.

different" from the strong-flavored and unattractive eggs which we all eat under compulsion or because we are still in ignorance of the real quality of the home-made article.

Does one reader object that he hasn't room to give his flock of fowls an outside run? An outside run is wholly unnecessary; the birds need never step foot outside the confines of the poultry house. This is one of the recent developments in poultry keeping, that when the flock is not kept for breeding but for egg-production alone the No-Yard system is quite as satisfactory, and gives even better results than where a considerable amount of ground is given to them to range over. This No-Yard system of keeping fowls is a wholly new idea to those who have been accustomed to see the fowls ranging all over the farm and garden and over the neighbors' gardens also. It works out perfectly, however, where the fowls are kept solely for egg-production, the birds being carried through one laying season only; being gradually killed for the fam-

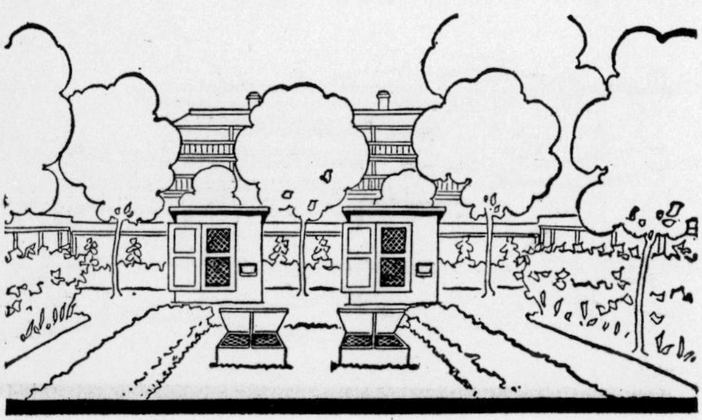

Same yard now paying a large part of the rent.

ily table or sold off to market in the late summer, and a new stock of laying pullets being installed in the house each fall. The flock is fed for eggs and lays eggs, and late in the summer any that have escaped the family's growing appetite for fresh killed fowl are shipped to market alive in time to clean and white-wash the house, making it ready for the new flock of pullets in October.

Does another reader object that he sends his family away to the seashore or the old home in the country directly after the schools close in June, and that he does not care to have a flock of fowls on his hands through the summer? The birds that are left on hand the last of June can be closed out to the hen-cart man, at a price closely approximating the first cost of the pullets, the very day before the wife and children flit from the home nest. Here is one illustration:—In the fall an acquaintance purchased a flock of twenty mixed pullets for twenty dollars and installed them in a small house which

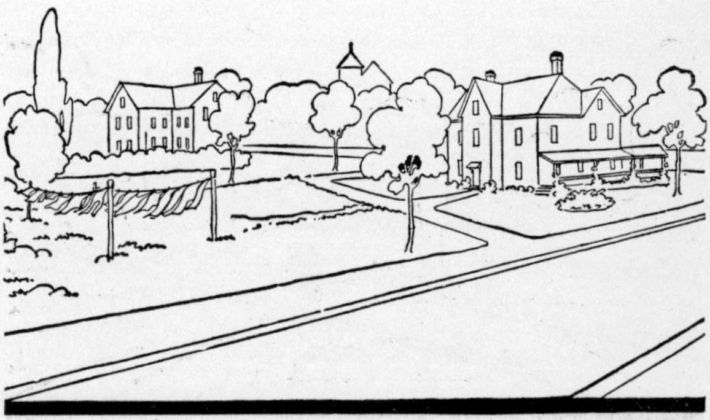

A vacant lot adjoining a village home. The taxes were heavy and the income nothing.

he had built of lumber from old packing cases in his back yard. From that date to July 7th following, he paid $19.50 for their feed; total capital and expense $39.50. During this period he sold to the grocer and used in his family eggs to the value of $80.89; the eggs used by the family being credited at the market prices of the time.

On July 7th, the following year, he moved his family into the country, to their summer home, and sold the hens to a hen-cart man for $10.12, making a total for eggs and hens sold of $91.01. Deducting the cost of feed bought and pullets we have $51.51 net profit on an investment of $20.00. Over and above that was the great satisfaction of having an abundance of eggs fresh from the nests for the family table.

An illustration of the rapid growth in popularity of this family flock idea is found in the experience of a poultryman living just outside the city of Toronto. A friend living in the city, having a small back yard to his house, bought a

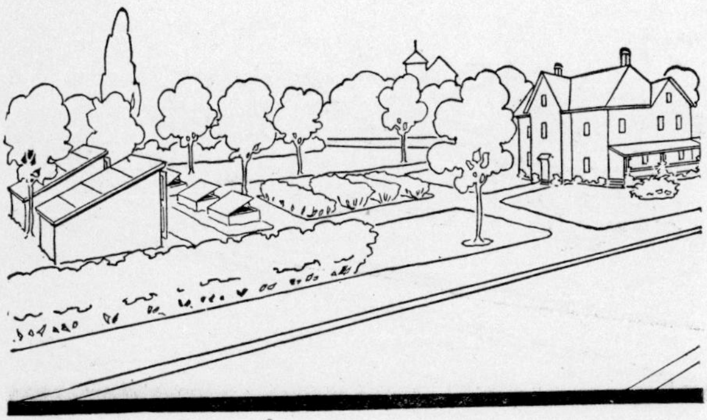

Same lot now pays the taxes and a nice income besides.

flock of ten pullets from him some half dozen years ago. This flock gave him an ample supply of fresh-laid eggs for home use and some to sell to his less fortunate friends and towards spring the family began eating a hen now and then as the appetite craved poultry-meat. When the family went away to the country for the summer the remaining birds were sold to the marketman. The city-man's friends envied him his good fortune, in his having fresh-laid eggs all through the fall, winter and spring and they got busy to provide the same blessing for their families, the net result being that our poultryman friend now has twenty-one families to whom he supplies a flock of ten, twelve or fifteen ready-to-lay pullets each October. All these families can credit to their backyard poultry plant greater health, wealth and happiness.

A man may feel that he cannot easily spare the time to feed and care for a flock of fowls. By the up-to-date methods of poultry keeping, a

Another suburban residence, the lady owner of which needed an income.

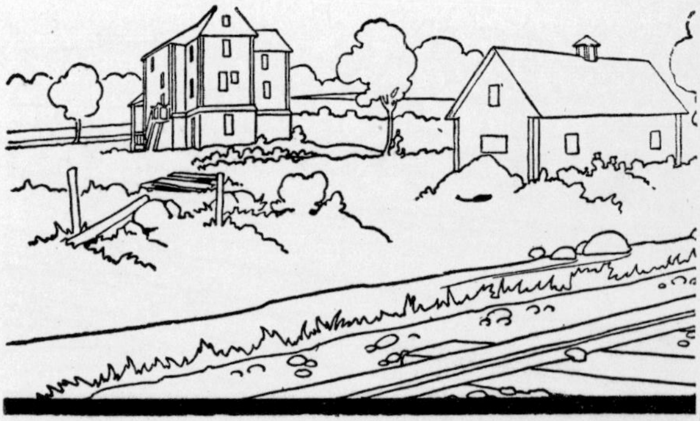

ten-year-old boy or girl can throw out to them the few handfuls of scratch feed in mid-afternoon, after coming from school. Then again it is no small advantage to a family to have an easy method of disposing of table and kitchen waste; the table and kitchen scraps of the ordinary family will half feed a flock of fowls, and gives them a much enjoyed variety of food. All the rest of the chores can be done in a few minutes after supper, the most important part of this last being the filling of the Egg Feed hoppers and the emptying of the drinking fountains so that the water shall not freeze in cold weather. In cold weather, too, the eggs should be gathered from the nests two or three times during the day to prevent their freezing.

Another man may say that he hasn't any chicken house. One suitable for a small flock can be quickly and cheaply built out of lumber from a few old boxes; if we want something more attractive, ready-made poultry houses that are

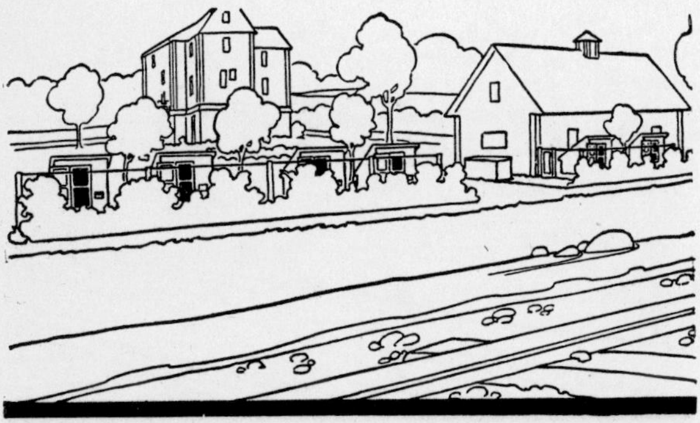

Same yard with poultry paying all expenses.

handy, convenient and attractive can be bought at moderate cost. These houses are shipped "knocked-down", can be quickly assembled and erected, and can be easily and quickly separated into several parts for removal if desired, as in the case of the family moving to another home. The No-Yard house is an excellent portable house, well adapted for a flock of a dozen to fifteen fowls. A description and illustration of this house seems desirable, and we give it on page 122.

It is not our intention in this chapter to enter into a discussion of the merits or demerits of any housing systems, but our experience, combined with thousands of successful poultrymen has proven to our satisfaction that in recommending the "open-front" house to the public we are advocating a system that has many advantages over any other.

A more complete outline of housing is given in the chapter by that title in this book, pages 117 to 128.

Old style poultry keeping.

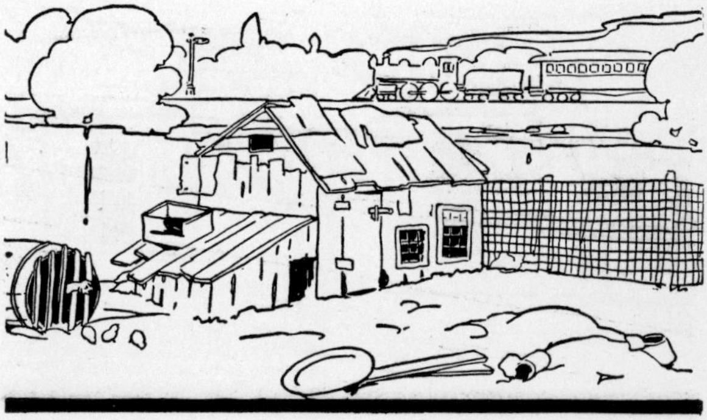

A good illustration of the especial point of this story has come to our notice. A young lady ot our acquaintance who had run down her health by too close application to office work in the city was ordered by her physician to eat two eggs each morning for her breakfast and take three eggs raw during the day. The difficulty of getting "dependably fresh" eggs suggested that she keep a small flock of fowls herself, and have home-grown eggs. Gaining her parents' permission to use a few square feet of the back of their lot for the purpose, she bought a "No-Yard" house, a flock of fifteen pullets and two bags of ready mixed feeds. The pullets laid splendidly all winter, not only giving her the fresh-laid eggs for her own use and a supply for the family, but she had a surplus to sell to the corner drug-store, where they sell for ten cents per dozen above the market price, and are used in egg-chocolate and other soft drinks.

This worked out so well that she has continued each year, fattening and selling off the birds in

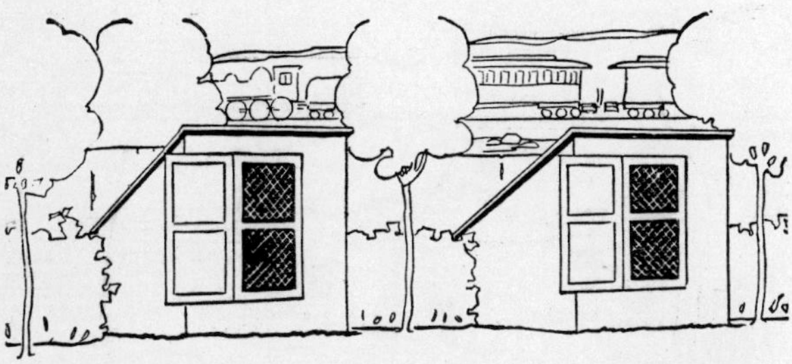

Same lot with up-to-date methods and No-Yard houses.

August and September, and buying new pullets again in the late fall to lay heavily during the season of high prices for eggs.

She pays her ten-year-old brother a small sum each week for doing the poultry work and says that she had not only achieved fresh-laid eggs for herself, but is making a good snug amount each year.

We have no sympathy with the "get-rich-quick" stories of $10 to $50 or $500 profit per hen in one year's time which are doing the rounds of the papers, solely for advertising purposes. We don't want our friends to get such greatly inflated figures into their minds, for they will be disappointed if they do. We do, however, want them to know that they can reduce their family living expenses by a substantial sum, by utilizing the table and kitchen waste and a small space in the back yard, both of which are not now used because of lack of opportunity. You can easily clear from $2.00 to $5.00 profit

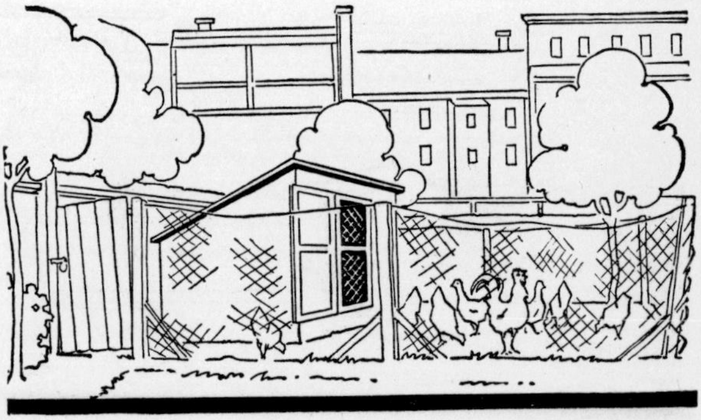

The picture that comes to many minds when back yard poultry-keeping is mentioned.

per year per hen on whatever number you can care for in your back yard, and the small amount of time spent with them will prove a recreation rather than a burden.

On a lot 50x50 feet in size there will be no difficulty in realizing a profit of from $50 to $500 a year on an investment of from $50 to $300. The old style method of poultry-keeping meant a lot of unsightly "shacks" and tumble-down yards, unending labor, and with results far from certain.

With our modern methods, of "no-yards" for the mature market egg birds and scientific feeding, the results are certain, the birds cannot get by without laying.

These statements sound pretty strong, but we are sure of our position.

Your garden will not suffer, in fact, both garden and lawn (if you have them) will be greatly improved by application of the droppings which are a most excellent fertilizer. The weeds from the garden, also the clippings from the lawn will

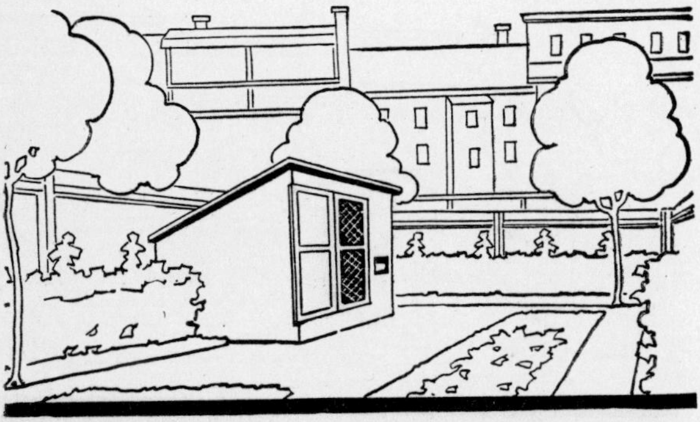

No-Yard system requires no male bird to disturb the neighborhood. It leaves ample space for a nice garden.

be greatly relished by the birds in confinement and less grain food will be eaten by them if they have the green food.

We well know that if these facts were realized by our friends more than double the poultry would be profitably kept and the family living expenses appreciably reduced. It takes years, however, to impress some of the most simple truths upon the minds of the doubters, meanwhile, the demand for eggs and poultry meat continues to increase much faster than the supply. Prices continue to soar and our doubting friends continue to rail at the beef trust, overlooking the fact that they have right at hand a powerful weapon against that organization, viz: shutting off a part of the trust's market by producing their own meat and eggs and by supplying their friends and neighbors. By so much they can decrease the trust's sales, and put a handsome profit in their own pockets.

So let the consumer of eggs and poultry be-

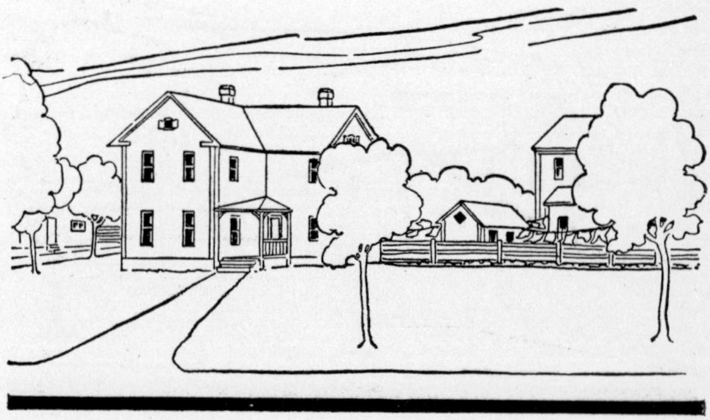

The young lady whose parents owned this estate was ordered by the physician to take fresh eggs daily.

come first the producer. There is money to be made, health to be gained and recreation and happiness will go hand in hand. While held in the city by the demands of the present day civilization, the back-to-the-farm yearning may be all but realized in the little back yard flock of poultry.

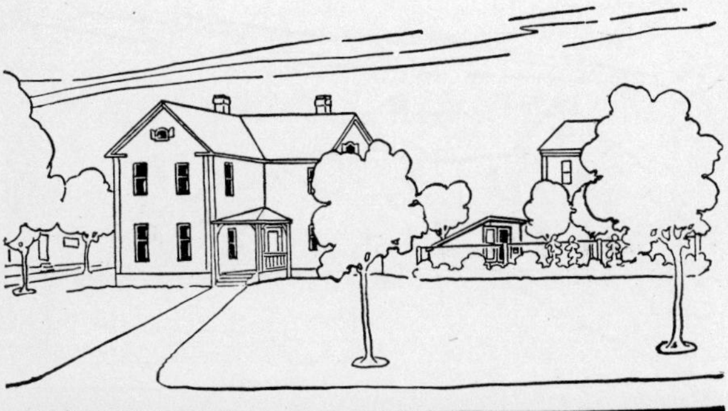

A poultry house was substituted for the unsightly view of a neighbor's back yard, and now fresh eggs are a regular morning delicacy for all the family.

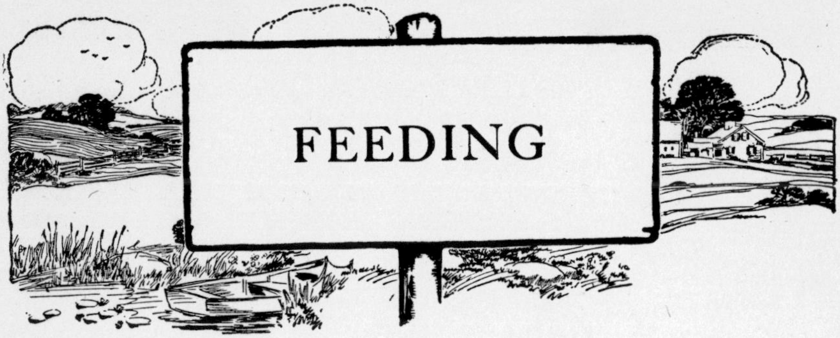

FEEDING

The success or failure of any poultry keeping undertaking really rests upon the skill of the feeder, for successful poultry keeping is only dependent upon two things, keeping the birds healthy and feeding them properly. We have shown the proper methods of housing and general care in other chapters and will try to give the outline of a safe feeding system or plan that will enable all to gain success with their birds.

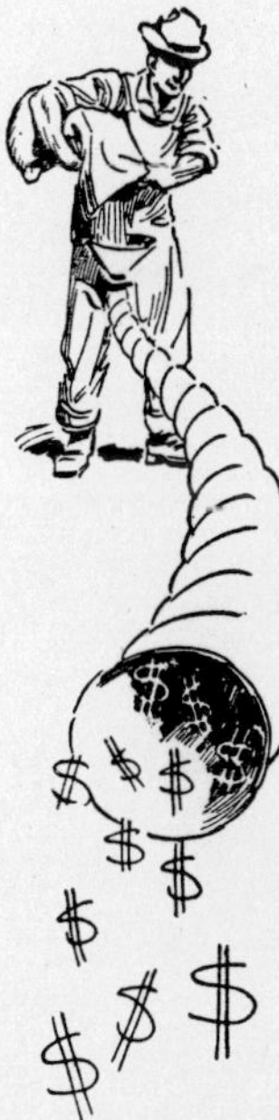

Heavy feeders make the money

One of the first principles to be always remembered is that your results are dependent upon liberal feeding and by liberal feeding we mean feeding all the birds can be coaxed to eat of the right materials, and we must consider feed as material and egg, poultry and breeding stock as the finished products.

There is no question that a newly hatched chicken is a delicate and tender object, keenly sensitive to neglect, but particularly sensitive to improper food. Properly fed and surrounded with half way right conditions as to temperature and air, he goes ahead at a wonderful rate—but improperly fed, he stands still and dies.

Practically speaking, his life horoscope is decided in the first ten days to three weeks of his existence. In this length of time, if he is a good husky fellow, he will eat from three to four cents' worth of feed.

If the chickens consumed the chick feed during the first month in their lives in the quantities they use when from three to five months of age, there might be a little excuse for looking for inexpensive rations, provided it did not imperil the lives of the youngsters, but when we consider that a pound of the best chick feed will put a chicken beyond the danger period, or up to three weeks of age, what excuse is there for the saving of a quarter of a cent a pound when it endangers the entire season's crop of producers? Really a poultryman would be better off in many instances if he paid double the price for the best chick feed, in preference to the gift of many of the feeds on the market.

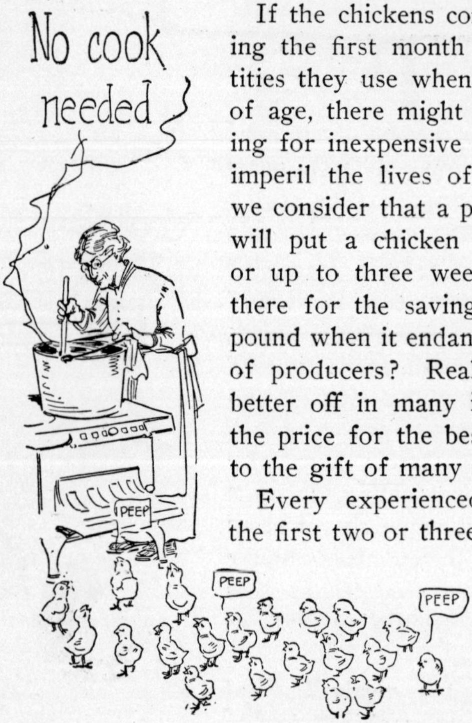

Every experienced poultryman realizes that the first two or three weeks is the crucial period in the lives of his chickens. Upon the health and thrift of the chickens during these few weeks depend the profits of the whole season, and of the year's business.

An all grain or vegetable diet is not natural to any age of poultry and it has been found highly beneficial to young chickens to combine a small amount of dried codfish or meat and add it to the cracked grains and seeds used in making up the chick feed ration. Certain preparations of codfish being used after having been put through a special preparatory process that eliminates all the fat, it supplies the newly hatched birds at the crucial age when most needed with animal protein, without the animal fat.

The yolk of the eggs not being fully absorbed until the chickens are ten days old and consisting largely of carbo-hydrates, furnishes all the materials of a fatty nature that is desirable. Thus if we add the commercial meat scraps containing more or less fat, there is very sure to be trouble, while in shredded codfish properly prepared not an atom of fat remains. We thus furnish just what the rapidly developing bodies require without any white diarrhoea—so fatal in some sections.

Cooking the food for chickens or grown poultry, only serves to render the starchy parts of the feed more digestible, but by so doing, throws the feeds out of balance, and while the chicks apparently thrive better for a few days, they later receive a set back that leaves them not so far ahead as the birds fed on raw foods from the start.

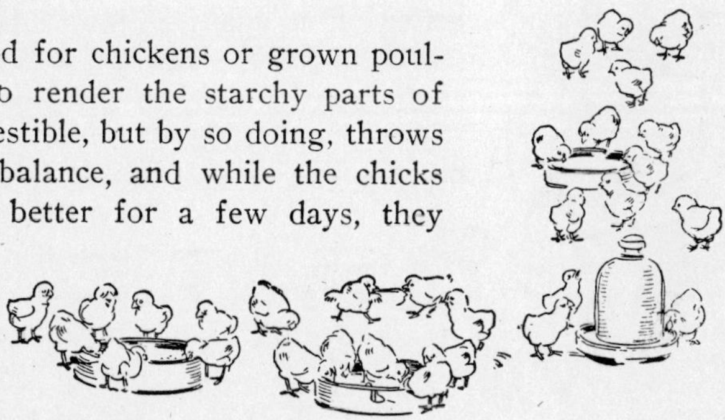

Nature put a Cook inside of them

With so much of our entire season's work and profits depending upon the chickens, realizing that they are going to be worth from one to two dollars each when grown, and that after they are three weeks of age very little mortality ensues—

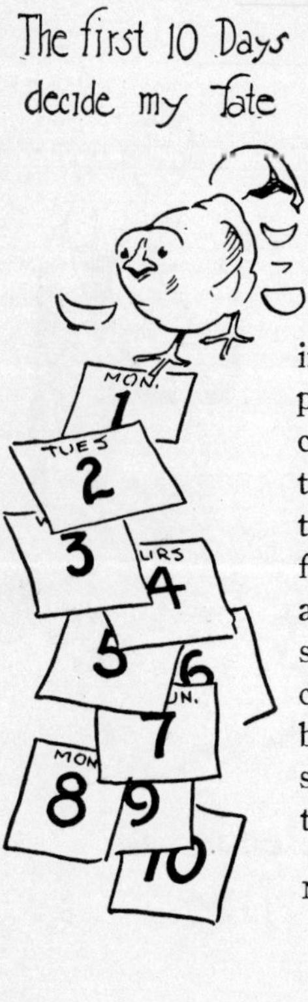
The first 10 Days
decide my fate
MON.
1
TUES
2
3
4
5
6
7
MON
8
9
10

it would seem folly to consider any feed for them but the BEST and most nourishing rations.

A coarser chick feed may be fed after the chicks reach three weeks of age, being fed in connection with Growing Feed. If the very highest perfection of development is desired with your birds, give alternate feeds of the best fine chick and of a coarser chick feed until the birds are eight weeks of age. Keep the Growing Feed continually before them. Remember that stuffing the birds to their limit, studying their habits and whims, all with the idea of getting more food into them by increasing their early growing habits, is a successful poultryman's aim. If you get a two-pound chicken at eight weeks of age, instead of ten or twelve weeks' time, you have gained from one to two weeks' feed, and the chances are from five to ten cents per pound in the selling value, as the market declines very rapidly during the spring and early summer months, and if your chickens are not in the market any earlier or better than the one thousand other poultrymen shipping to the same market you are not going to receive any better prices than they get.

NINE-TENTHS OF THE CHICKENS HATCHED DO NOT GET ENOUGH TO EAT.

Why so many chickens are hatched, and so few really fed, is a great problem, but we think that the improper feeding and poor quality of unbalanced rations are largely responsible, for all will recognize the fact that most of the teachings of ten years ago,—and in many cases of today,—are to keep your chickens "on edge", or hungry all the time.

Your chickens should never be hungry, as the term is generally understood. HUNGRY BIRDS ARE NOT GROWING.

Almost without exception in all other forms of bird and animal life the growing period is the fattening period of life. In other words, the birds or animals carry more fat on them during this than any other time of their lives, and in the face of this, the old teaching told us to "keep them hungry." Is it any wonder that the hens did not lay, that the youngsters did not get to standard weight, or that poultry keeping did not pay?

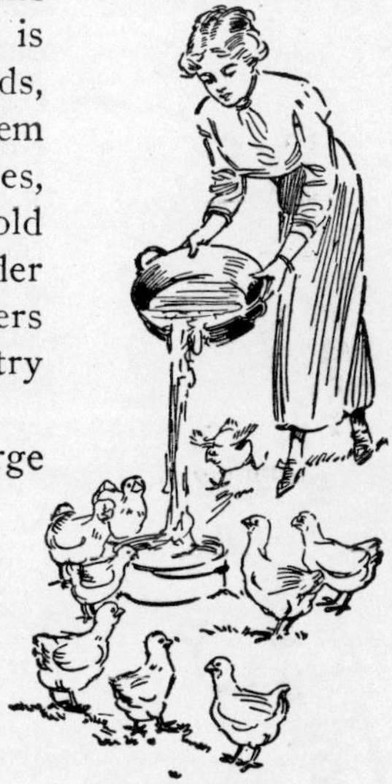

Change of Diet

Hen-reared chickens, when running at large with the mother hen, are fed a continuous stream of bugs, worms, grains, seeds and grasshoppers, from daylight to dark. There is no interval of fasting; only brief warm-up recesses or naps; the entire day is spent in trying to "fill up." The feeding system we advocate gives these same conditions. After the chickens are ten days to two weeks old provide them with ground Growing Feed which furnishes them with a continuous ration which should be made up of a happy combination of the strongest and richest grains and meat food ground together in the most appetizing form for the chickens to so please their palates that they will stuff themselves from one week's end to the other, and grow evenly and rapidly into highly developed pullets, cockerels, or capons, in one-third less time than they would under any other system.

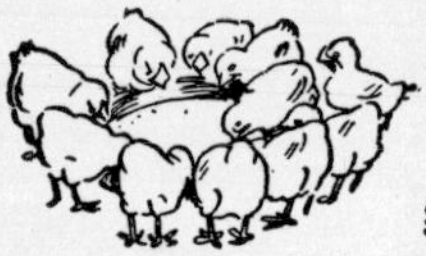

Upon a properly balanced Growing Feed ration, cockerels reach ten and twelve pounds weight in six months, thus representing a growth in each day of their lives equal to two-thirds of their entire weight when hatched into this cold, hard world.

YES

? $?

NO

To make this growth, conditions must be right, and the feed must be rich, abundant, and always within reach. It must also be present in a form that is not only palatable to the growing chickens, but in such form as will digest most economically and completely. Now it is easy to see that wet food cannot be kept before them constantly and remain sweet.

Poultry rations that have been in use in the past for growing stock are too restricted, and do not fully nourish all parts of the rapidly growing system, and some of the chickens break down at all ages.

Fanciers recognize as an almost universal fact that late hatches or summer chickens are the best colored and the best formed of any of their broods, and their problem has been getting them to standard size in season for the winter shows.

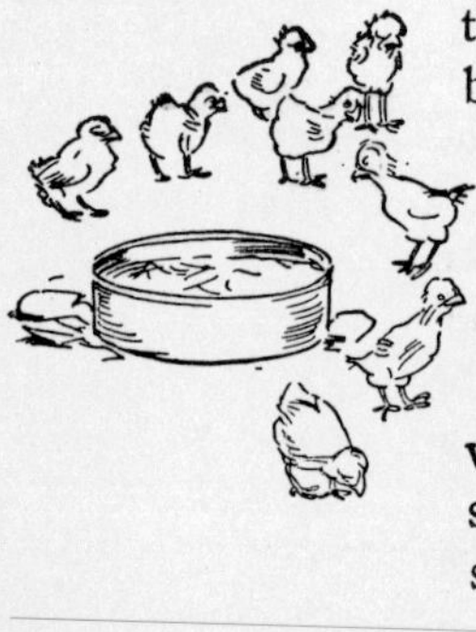

This rapid growth and full development is just what a properly prepared Growing Feed will do, giving a wide variety to feed upon, and so fully nourishing every part of the growing stock that they are always in good form and well feathered with unlimited stamina that will reproduce itself in next season's breeding pen with even better and greater strength.

Added to this is the big item of saved labor over the expenditure of time in preparing and "serving" wet mash mixtures.

This enormous saving of time and food is not at the expense of any vital function, but rather the reverse, for the stock will rapidly increase in strength and vitality under this treatment, and after you try it a season you will find your old stock one to two pounds heavier, and your pullets laying a month earlier.

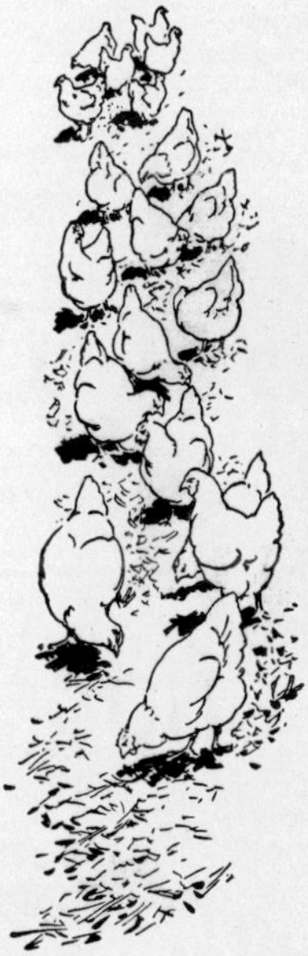

Give your chickens a chance to show you how skillfully you did your mating last season, and the only way you can do so, is to feed them to the limit.

Remember, full fed chickens are paying chicks.

The Scratch Feed should be compounded to balance the Egg Feed and should always be very carefully screened and composed of a combination of the very best and sweetest grains and seeds, which pleases the taste of the hen and at the same time keeps her everlastingly scratching. The exercise she gets in this way increases her activity, develops the muscles and blood vessels, helps digestion and circulation, reddens the comb, and assists in a general way to strengthen all the functions of the body. A scratching hen is like a whistling boy or a singing girl—always happy, and generally busy. We believe in giving poultry plenty to do.

A variety of grains more fully nourishes the

many complicated parts of the bird's anatomy, and results in larger and stronger fowl with increased vitality. When confined to a restricted ration, young stock do not fill out as well; are more subject to disease, and fail to reach the size that they would attain if fed liberally upon a carefully balanced mixture. Laying hens are more subject to disease, acquire pernicious habits of egg eating, feather pulling, etc., simply as a result of the natural craving of an appetite unsatisfied. Given a carefully balanced ration, they acquire none of these bad habits and show their appreciation in full baskets of fertile eggs throughout the year.

Study to stuff the hens during short feeding Hours.

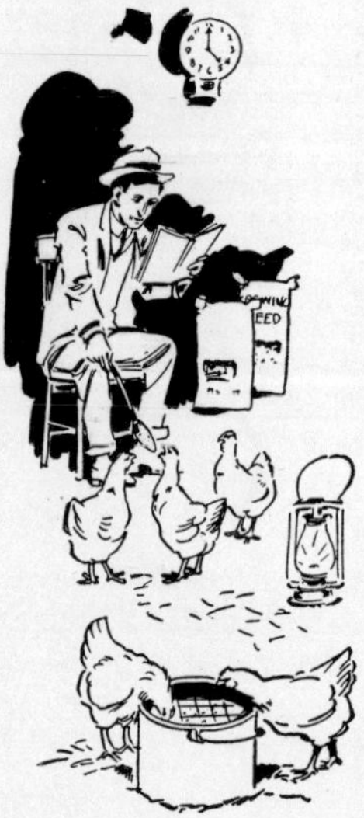

For instance, buckwheat in itself is one of the best egg producers on the entire list of grains, but if fed to excess, and without other grains to counteract the tendency, produces eggs with very pale yolks.

Wheat is an excellent egg producer, but fed too freely reduces the strength of the germs and vitality of the chickens hatched.

Nothing but long experience with the birds gives this information, and makes it possible to counteract the weak features of each ingredient with the strong features in some other material.

An egg is the product of a very wonderfully developed and sensitive organism, containing the nucleus of undeveloped germs for generations upon generations to come. This action of the generative organs is a very heavy drain upon the hen's system; nothing parallels it in Nature. A milch cow is an approach, but she is not drawing on her reproductive organs as often as in nature, but the hen has, by man's careful manipulation, increased her reproductive capacity many times since becoming a servant of mankind.

This saps her vitality and we can only hope to keep her wonderfully made machinery in operation without interruption or breakdown by placing within her reach an abundance of such food as she likes, without having any "stop-watch" on her to tell when she has eaten enough.

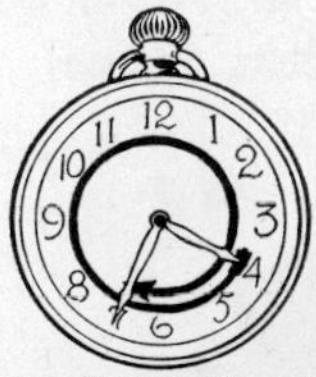

15 FEEDING HOURS IN SUMMER AGAINST

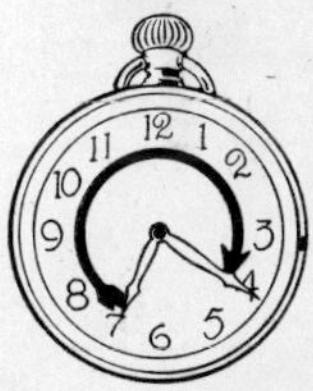

9 FEEDING HOURS IN WINTER

Instead of being "used up" with that tired feeling in the spring season when we want strong eggs for hatching purposes, she is steadily producing eggs that hatch well, and chickens that live well. She skips all the ailments and diseases caused by improper feeding, and continues to contribute to the prosperity of her owner for the full twelve months of the year.

Scratch Feeds are usually made the dump of refuse grains that cannot be sold in the open market, and when making comparisons with prices of feed keep in mind that every kernel of grain in your mixture should be sweet, and that they contain no sweepings or weed seed.

For the best results in egg production we recommend one or two Feeders containing Egg Feed constantly before the birds, and a feed of Scratch Feed in litter an hour or two before roost time at night. This gives an opportunity to fill up at the time of day when Nature warns them that they need a full crop to last them until morning. They do not have a chance to gorge themselves early in the day and then dope around, but are always on the move between feed hopper and litter looking for some of last evening's remnants, and have no time to line up in the sunlight as wet-mash fed hens are prone to do on a cold winter day after a hot mash in the morning.

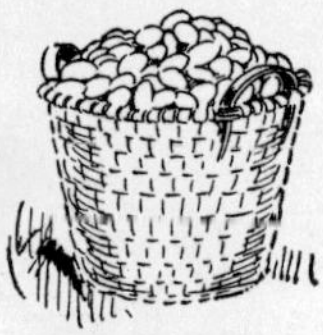

Years ago a wise old poultryman said, "There's more in the feed than in the breed," and he was certainly right. We would say that it is all in the feed. Perhaps that would be too strong a statement, but certainly all will admit that the breed counts for very little, or nothing, without the feed. The best bred hens cannot—and will not—lay if not fed, and the poorest scrub will lay quite plentifully if properly fed. Feed has more to do with the paying end of a poultry plant than anything else, and the only feed that is cheap is the feed that produces results.

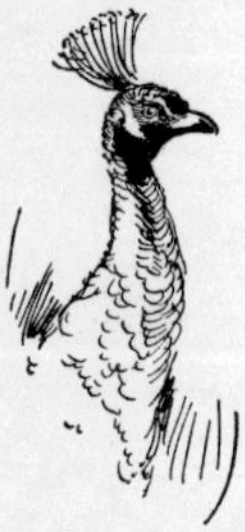

Results in the Egg basket rather than beauty of bird, are what we are seeking.

A properly compounded Egg Feed always will produce eggs at a lower cost per hen than any other feed. After carefully experimenting for years we have demonstrated that egg eating, feather pulling, going broody, getting over-fat, and "going light" may be—and are—largely overcome by its use.

These points should be given constant and careful consideration, and the requirements followed out regardless of the cost of the proper materials.

A fluctuating grain market does not mean that high priced ingredients necessary to the proper balancing of feeds be left out of these mixtures;

this would be poor economy. A proper Egg Feed should give you the results you are looking for every day in the year.

The proper blending of ingredients is as important as to have the proper materials. Feeding your birds the right materials in the wrong proportions will just as surely throw them out of condition, resulting in a train of ill success, infertile eggs, weak chickens and low vitality among your stock, as feeding the wrong materials.

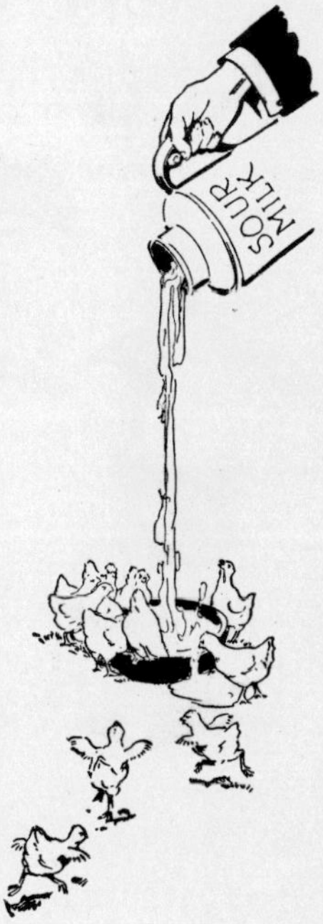

In purchasing feeds, watch your protein analysis. A low protein feed at a low price costs you more per feeding value than a high protein feed at a much higher price, and we emphasize, —THIS PROTEIN MUST BE *ANIMAL* PROTEIN; NOT *VEGETABLE* PROTEIN.

Formulas have been put out by various experiment stations embodying the use of vegetable protein in combination with animal protein, thereby lessening the cost over some rations which depend upon animal protein altogether. These vegetable protein rations, while good, will not maintain the highest volume of efficiency, nor will they maintain the birds in the best of health. In confirmation of this we would refer you to the report of the Massachusetts Agricultural Experiment Station, Bulletin No. 122, March 1908.

> "'For laying hens the rations containing animal food proved superior to others in which all the organic matter was derived from vegetable sources,

* * * * * It appears also that while a cheaper vegetable food ration can sometimes be made to equal or surpass in efficiency a ration containing animal food by supplementing it with suitable mineral matter, there are plain limitations to its economical use. For laying hens, some animal food appears necessary for continued good results.'

Judging from our own results and from those obtained by Wheeler, it seems safe to conclude that animal albuminoids as measured by production possess a much higher degree of efficiency than those derived from vegetable materials."

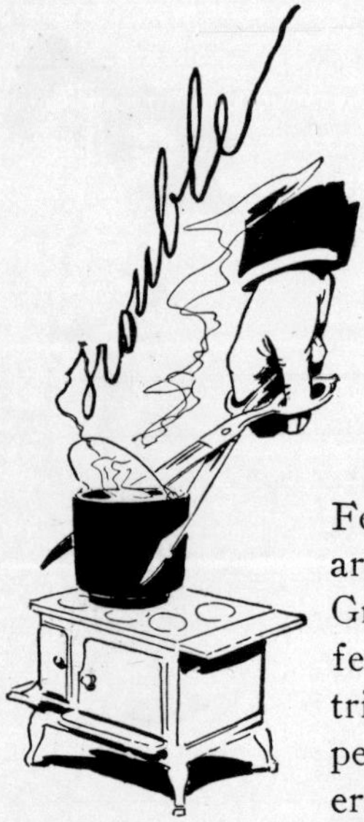

Cut out the hot Mash
It spells TROUBLE

Start your pullets on a ration of Growing Feed and Egg Feed, half of each, when they are about one month from laying, dropping the Growing Feed as they begin to lay. Keep the feed in one or more hoppers, boxes or other contrivances, in light, easily accessible parts of the pen, and do not let them go empty. Feed a liberal quantity of Scratch Feed about an hour before they go to roost in litter, inducing them to scratch freely. Encourage them to eat liberally of the Egg Feed, at least as much in bulk as of the Scratch Feed, cutting down the Scratch Feed until this is brought about, but getting every ounce of feed into them you can, and your egg basket will show the results we all look for. Egg Feed and Scratch Feed make a complete balanced ration, but if you have cabbage or clover it is well enough to feed it, although the Dry-Mash itself should contain a liberal amount of Alfalfa. Simply furnish shells, grit, and an ample supply of water in addition.

In the newer settled portions of the country we find a disposition to relax all mash feeding as soon as the grass comes in the spring, the owners knowing that the hens always lay at this season of the year anyway.

They overlook the fact that the hens now lay by Nature's bidding and in many instances take it out of their bodies in reducing their fat, depending upon their resting period in raising a flock of chickens to restore them to natural weight.

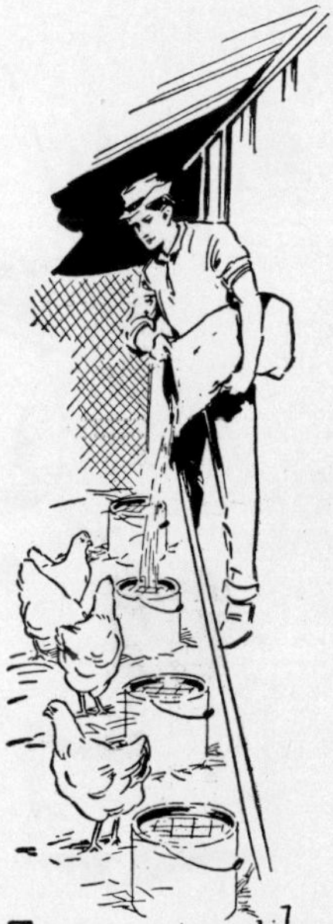

Eggs steadily increasing in price.

Now the owner perhaps does not wish to have them incubate and "breaks them up" and starts them laying again, they lay a short litter and start setting again. When broken up a second time they are very likely to hold off from laying for a considerable time, as not being fed upon a rich ration they have little incentive to lay and if running at large they are too busy seeking grasshoppers and insects to think much of laying.

If the owners of these birds would keep up their winter feeding right through the year, they would get heavy egg records all summer and fall and double their profits over their present system. Hens are gluttons, they produce from five to ten times their weight each year in eggs if fed properly. Your profits depend upon their eating. Increase your profits by increasing the eating process.

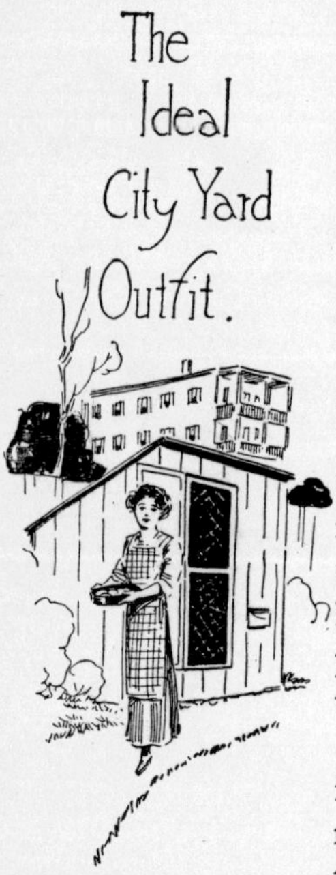

To get the maximum number of eggs from the number of birds, confine them in small lots of from 15 to 30, allowing them three or four square feet floor space to each bird. See that they get a liberal amount of pure air through one opening in the south side at all times, night and day, winter and summer. Do not let them out of the house from the time they go into it in the fall until they go to market the next fall. Feed as directed above and you will get more eggs than ever before.

We cannot tell you why, and do not attempt to reason it out. We can only state that we have found more eggs and at a less cost result when no yard was used with this system of feeding. This very materially reduces the expense of constructing and maintaining a poultry plant, leaves much more room for the growing chickens, or doubles the number of birds kept on an acre of land, and works a wonderful advantage when the pullets are bought each season, and we have only words of praise for, the system.

Think of the labor saved! Think of the capital saved! Think of the worry saved! One man's labor alone will care for 2,500 birds on this system. If you have an empty house or two, buy a lot of mixed pullets, try out this system, and tell us if you have not opened a way to commercial poultry keeping on a business basis.

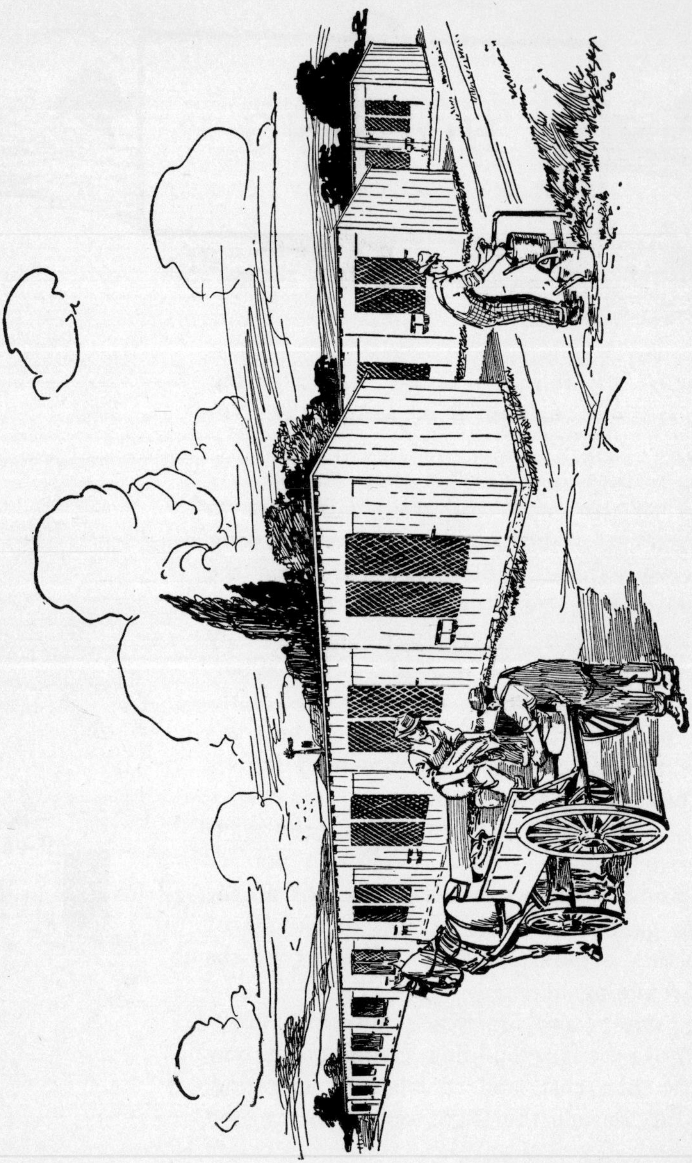

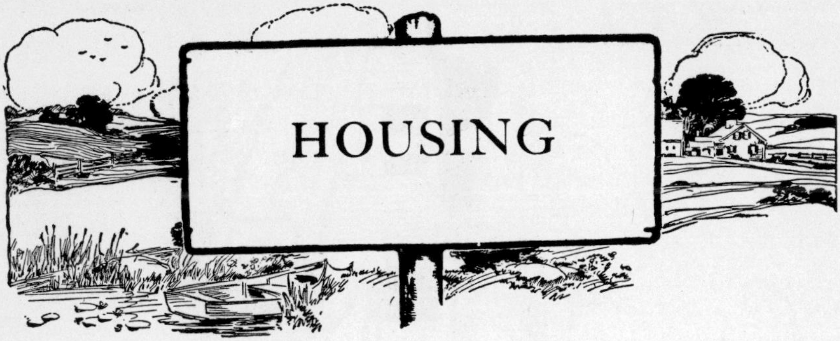

HOUSING

THOUSANDS of families would start keeping poultry if they realized how simple the No-Yard system really is.

When poultry is suggested they immediately think of all the detail and trouble incident to raising chickens,—the annoyance of the crowing of the cocks, the unsightly back yard, and the neighbors' protests in general.

It is our purpose here to show that not only can poultry be kept in a neat and tidy manner, but that the original outlay may be almost nothing if one is a little handy with tools and has the time to put into the construction of houses out of boxes or waste lumber.

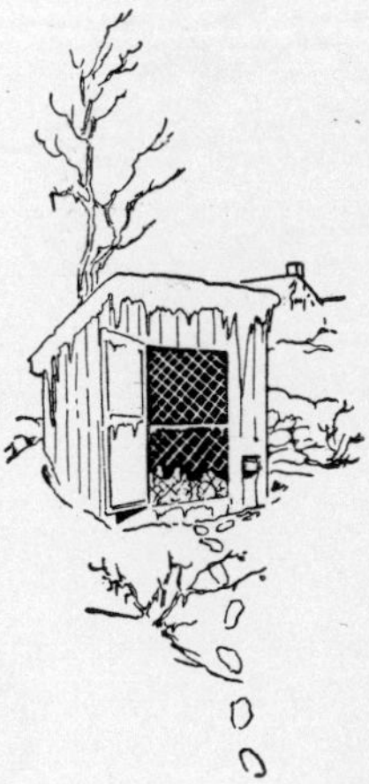

Pages and volumes of matter have been written regarding shape, sizes and styles of poultry houses, and the subject is well worthy of all the attention paid to it. The success or failure of many plants is determined at the outset by the style of building adopted.

Some writers and practical poultrymen advocate and use the long building, claiming economy in construction cost, and of labor in operating.

We will concede the slight saving in the cost

of construction, but when considered as a twelve months' proposition, we know that houses on the colony plan will give much better returns on the capital invested.

We must consider the bird's comfort twelve months in the year, and what would seemingly be best for a blowy January day would be stifling on a hot day in July.

What would serve to the best purposes the comfort of the bird in August would be altogether too exposed in December. Windows are out of the question, as they make a very hot building when the sun is shining and equally cold quarters after dark, bringing two extremes of temperature during a single day, a shock no bird can stand, and keep in condition.

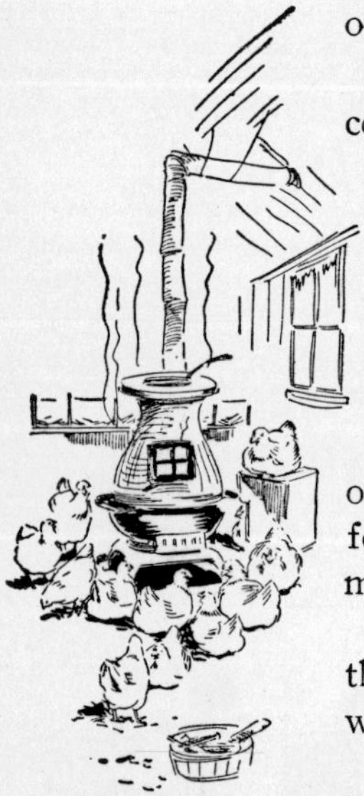

Nothing doing on the nests.

We have tried about every size, style and type of building that has been advocated, and have found that the small portable building brings the most uniform success to all users.

These houses make the birds comfortable in the hottest day in summer, or the coldest day in winter, and require practically no attention.

Poultry, and in fact everything wearing feathers, are of course, creatures of the air, and the importance of right air conditions surrounding the birds is recognized as of paramount importance in keeping the birds in health.

Poultry in health, properly fed, produce remarkable results; in fact, a hen working along smoothly is the greatest producer in the animal kingdom.

This may seem a broad statement, but think

of it! In twelve months' time she will produce from five to ten times her weight in eggs, and that means practically five to ten times her weight in flesh.

Thus, our study must be to maintain her henship in the most perfect health.

The best way to cure sickness is to prevent it. Nine-tenths of really bad poultry diseases originate from bad air, and can all be prevented by right air conditions.

Your birds will never have influenza, colds, roup, catarrh, canker or chicken pox if always surrounded with proper air.

Now to produce the right air conditions we must carefully study the shape and diagram of our house.

The main part to consider is that one-third of the south side shall be open to the weather in all climates and under all conditions, and that the opening be covered with one-inch wire netting on the front of the door, and that the opening be equally distant from each side of the pen and from the roof and bottom of the pen.

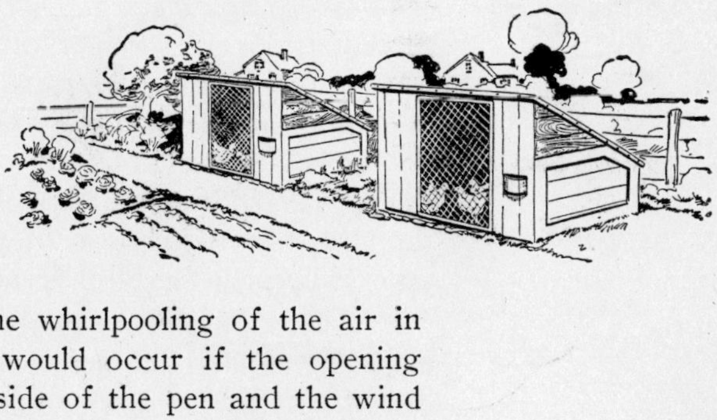

This prevents the whirlpooling of the air in the house, which would occur if the opening were next to one side of the pen and the wind was blowing against the front of the house from an angle.

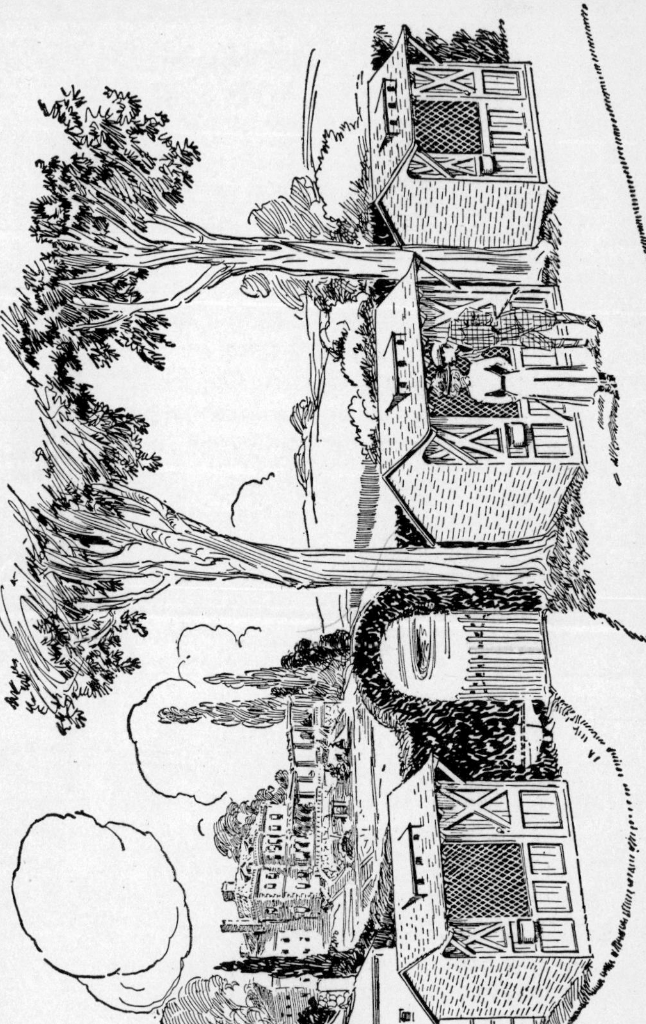

As to the exact form of the house, almost any size or plan seems efficient so long as the south side opening is the only one in the pen, and is as described.

Set the building up on posts when it arrives, or if the ground is frozen too hard to make it possible to dig post holes, simply set it on four corner stones or wooden blocks, scraping off the snow and filling the house in six inches to a foot above the bottom edge of the siding with fairly dry sand or gravel. If the ground is not frozen, set up on four corner posts, fill in with earth and gravel, and bank up the outside two or three inches above the lower edge of the house. Put six inches to a foot of good litter on top of the sand or gravel. Leave the cloth door open every day, unless the storm is coming from the south, (assuming that your building faces the south), and you are ready for your live stock.

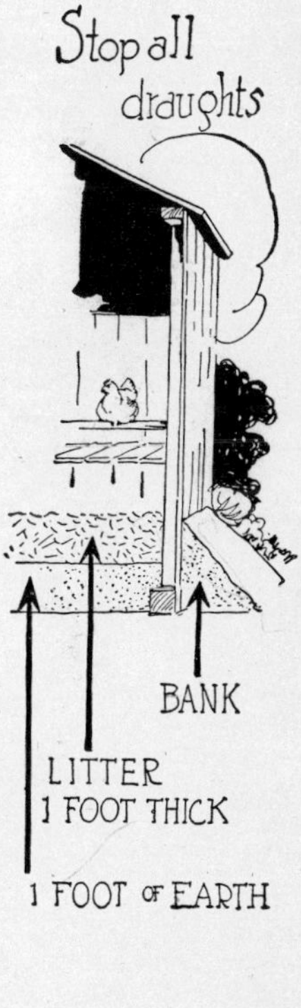

Improper housing is one of the things that figures strongly against profitable poultry.

In climates as severe as New England we recommend that not less than one-third of the entire south surface of the house be constructed of wire only, with a light frame covered with cheese cloth or waterproof sheeting, for use on nights when the temperature ranges below zero; or for use during the driving storms when the house is very narrow so that storms beat in onto the birds on their roosts. At other times, day and night, cloth doors should be kept fastened back, so as to give a free circulation of air.

For climates less severe than New England,

ranging to summer conditions, we should modify this plan only by increasing the amount of wire on the south side.

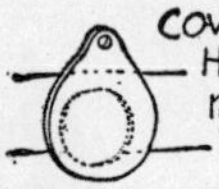

Cover to Hole over nest

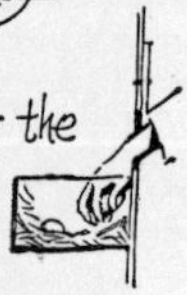

Removing the eggs

For southern states, California and other mild climates of the same character, we should recommend that the entire south side of the building be constructed of wire only, without any cloth whatever.

We should aim to err in the direction of always giving the birds more air, if the slightest doubt remains in our minds on that point. This method of housing will make a world of difference in the health of your flock.

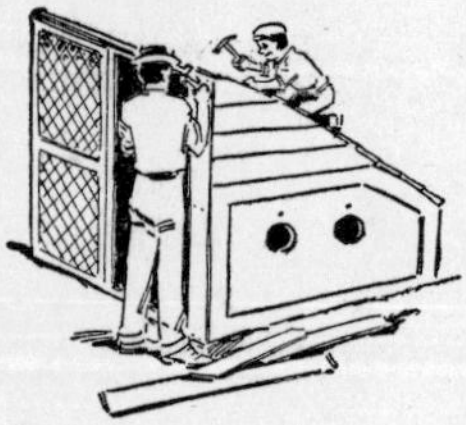

Putting on the sides and roof.

We especially recommend the "No-Yard" house shown on page 114.

This "No-Yard" poultry house is 6 feet wide, 8 feet deep, 6½ feet high at the front and 4 feet high at the back. The back and two sides are built of heavy, high-grade matched flooring, tongued and grooved and solidly put together so that it is impossible for air to enter at any point. The front is built of the same material and has two doors opening in opposite directions, one inside and the other outside. The inner door is covered with one-inch galvanized diamond-mesh wire that serves to confine the hens to the house and at the same time exclude objectionable intruders. The outer door is covered with waterproof cloth, and will be found necessary only in case of a severe storm, when it will effectually

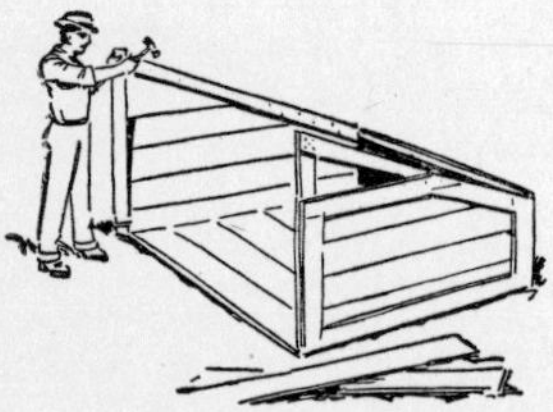

Putting in roof supports after side of piano box is removed

exclude the rain or snow and at the same time permit a free circulation of pure air. The roof is constructed of heavy one-inch matched lumber, reinforced around the four sides and down the center by wide strips of the same material. The entire roof is covered by heavy No. 27 galvanized steel that makes it impervious to rain, snow and wind. When the house is "set-up" it is tightly held together by galvanized steel corner pieces and with the overhanging edges of the roof it is "absolutely waterproof."

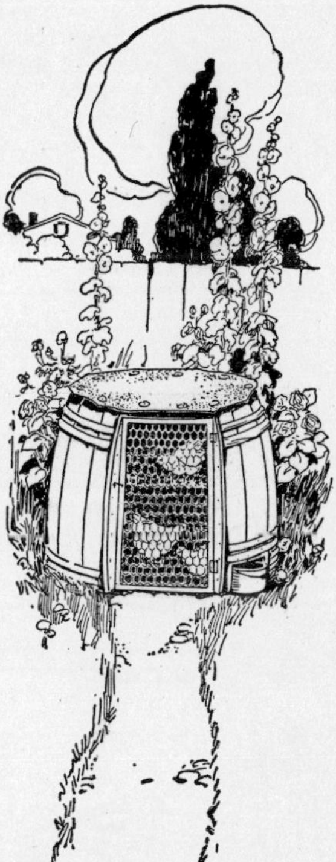

This inexpensive outfit can be made attractive.

The illustration of the interior shows two heavy roosts six feet long complete with a dropping board. The location of these roosts makes it absolutely impossible for draughts to strike the fowl from any direction. The laying box hung on the side has three compartments that are arranged in the most practical manner, that permit the hens to lay their eggs in comfort. The roosts, dropping board and laying box are all easily removed for cleansing.

It will be noted that the arrangement of the interior fixtures in this house leaves the entire floor space at the disposal of the hens for scratching and allows for the accommodation of its maximum capacity.

Such a house can be purchased and shipped "knocked-down" of the supply houses at a price ranging from $25.00 to $30.00, or if second-hand lumber can be had at reasonable prices the same building can be put up at from eight to fifteen dollars, using roofing paper for covering the cracks in the sides, back and roof.

Of course, this price does not include the labor, as we are assuming that the reader is to build it himself.

A very satisfactory and acceptable house may be improvised from a crockery barrel by sawing off about three of the staves, as illustrated, a door put in place, and water and feed provided.

This should not cost over 50c. to $1.00, and makes quite a satisfactory residence for a family of five pullets, and you can safely count on three or five eggs per day with half the rations coming from the waste of the table.

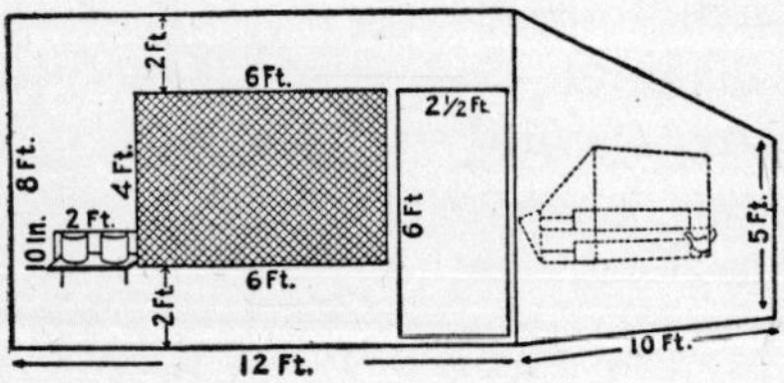

Another very popular and inexpensive house can be made of a piano box and when completed makes a house for six to eight pullets, and will not cost over $3.00 to $4.00.

We should prefer the houses without floors, and built on this plan there will be enough lumber in the original box to build the entire building.

Make the most of the room by building shelves eighteen inches by two feet in width, about two feet above the height of the litter on the floor. Keep water dishes, nests, feed dishes and shell and grit boxes on these shelves, thus giving every bit of floor space to the birds to scratch over.

The same general interior plan can be preserved and a more imposing outside struc-

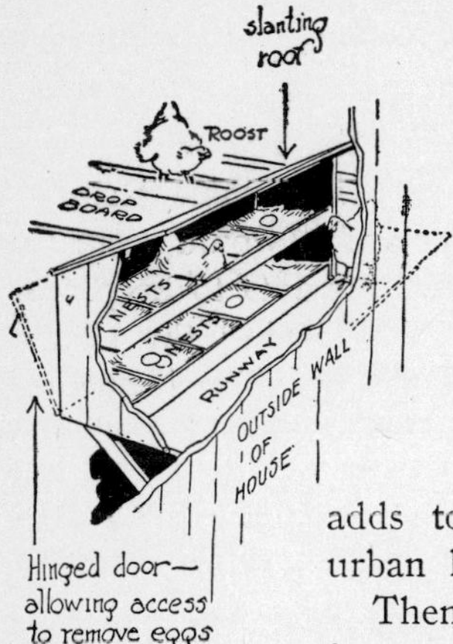

ture constructed on the lines shown on page —. This building can be varied in every way to match the architecture of the main building. Painted and surrounded with shrubbery or quick growing vines it usually adds to the charm of suburban life.

Then again some would-be poultrymen think of the long building they see on the large poultry farms, and really keep out of the business because of the unsightliness of the long, low buildings, unrelieved by any change or variation in design.

The "No-Yard" plan can readily be made to fit the landscape architect's scheme by grouping the buildings upon the rises among the trees in such a manner as is shown on page 120.

If you are determined to build a long house, we urge that you build it with absolutely no doors between pens, with tight board partitions running to the roof, and made as tight as building paper and boards can make them, the pens to be cared for entirely from the front just as in the "No-Yard" house.

Another very good plan is a house ten by twelve feet in size for thirty or forty birds.

This house will cost from $25.00 to $50.00 and is more adapted to poultry farms than to back yards, as its increased size renders it rather a permanent building, while the smaller ones can be easily constructed on the portable plan.

From the foregoing plans it would seem that almost anybody who really wants to keep poultry, who is interested in keeping the cost of living down, might start now. The business is simplicity itself when the No-Yard plan is adopted.

This method of housing and caring for the birds opens up the possibilities of the business. In the case of the farmer's boy desiring more spending money, he can build a house in most any out-of-the-way spot, provided the land is dry, and he never need worry about the hens getting out of their yard and into the garden or doing other mischief while he is away at school. By increasing the number kept, he can make enough money to take him through college, at the same time learning principles of business that will prove of inestimable value to him in later life.

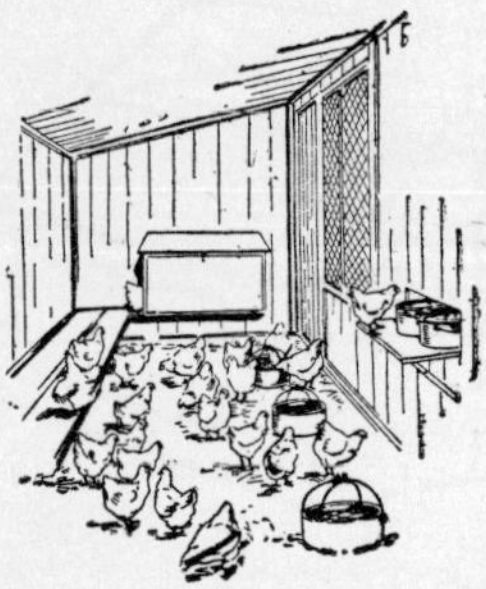

For the farmer, desiring to make use of every ounce of fertilizer and every foot of space upon his farm, this system appeals most strongly; in fact, it is the only system that gives him absolute control over the birds; preserves all the fertilizing value of the droppings, and enables him to make use of his land to the best advantage. He will find that if he invests $100, $500, or $1,000 in poultry and poultry building, follows the simple suggestions in this book, it will return him more profit than four times the money invested in any other branch of farm work and his returns are immediate and continuous.

The housewife also may provide herself and home with many luxuries and spending money, rendering herself in a measure independent of the head of the house. The business will be found particularly adapted to women desiring to retain their independence, or those on whom the burden of life rests heavily with others dependent upon them. The maternal instinct, prominent in women, and practically unknown to men, makes them much more successful in rearing chickens, and we must invariably take off our hats to them in this line.

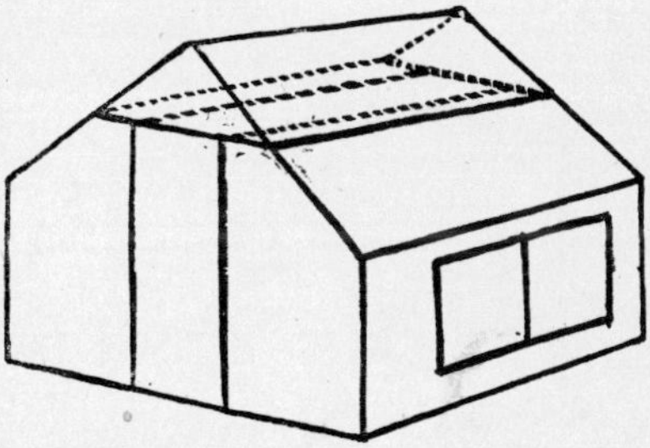

Back-yard poultry keepers have a great advantage in some ways over the more fortunate farmers that are farther away from market. We have frequently noticed that there is a constantly increasing demand for strictly fresh eggs, and the man or woman who takes up poultry keeping in the thickly settled communities may rest assured that the surplus eggs he has to dispose of will bring from 5 to 25 cents more per dozen than the wholesale prices.

With the "No-Yard System" these back yard and vacant lot plants are becoming much more common, as by this system no unsightly bare spot of land is left to mar the landscape.

No chickens being raised, no male birds are kept and the neighbors have no complaint to make of his early crowing.

It will be found in most cases that the table waste from an ordinary family will furnish nearly one-half the living for a dozen hens, and the waste and our feeds make an ideal combination for full egg production.

With the premium the neighbors so willingly pay for eggs "right out of the nest" and this saving in the feed cost, we are safe in saying that from $2.00 to $4.00 profit can be realized on each laying pullet.

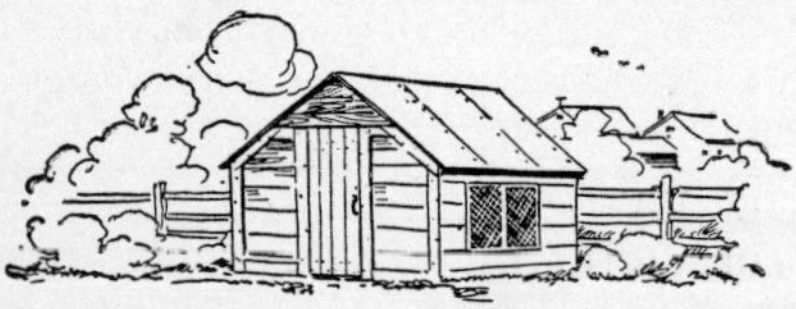

Not only are the profits assured, but the difference in flavor between the eggs gathered daily and the eggs to be obtained from the store will more than repay the care of the flock.

There is hardly a good-sized lot on which the owner or tenant may not make a profit of from $25 to $200 per year with a few minutes' time, night and morning, devoted to poultry keeping.

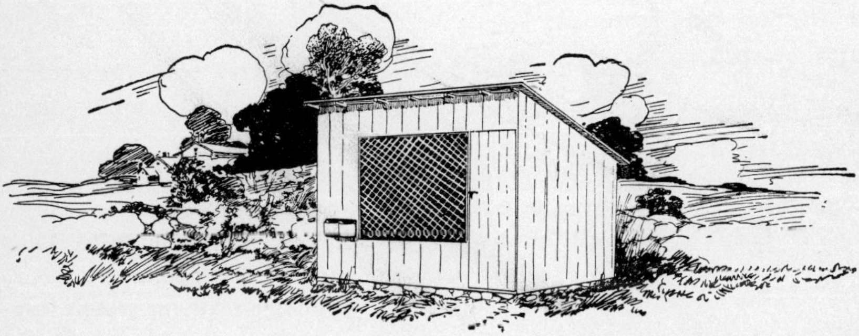

FOR
MY
SAKE
READ
THESE
DON'TS

We find there has been some confusion in the minds of readers and the poultry public regarding the advocacy of no yards for poultry.

We decidedly recommend large runs and free range for growing stock and breeding stock wherever possible, but with birds from which no stock is to be perpetuated—being used for the production of table eggs only,—the No-Yard System will be found to give much heavier egg yields and to require the minimum of care, room and expense.

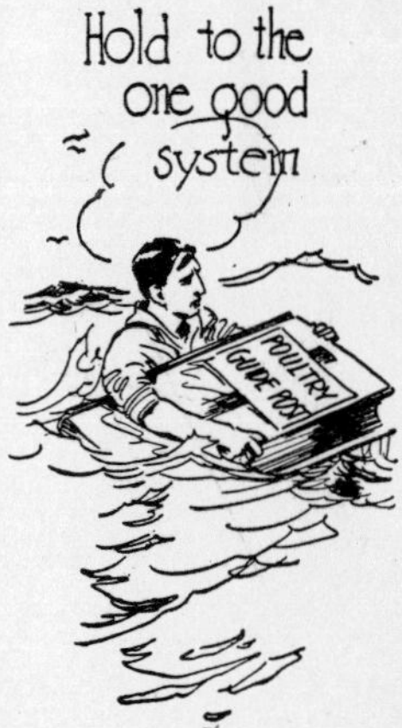
Hold to the one good system
POULTRY GUIDE POST

Breeding stock should not only have outdoor exercise 365 days in the year, but should have good sized yards and a much smaller number of females to the male than is usually provided throughout the country.

This system of feeding, housing, brooding and rearing has made success for thousands of poultry plants, and will for you if you will follow directions exactly. Do not, however, use a part of this system and expect best results. Use the whole system and be sure of results.

Do not institute into your plant a part of the system, mixing it with poultry paper suggestions, neighbors' advice and friends' criticisms. There is only one way to take a cold bath,—you cannot take it piece-meal; take it all over. Where this system is radically different from what you have been practising, try it in a whole-hearted manner, just as we outline it,—in one or two flocks only if you wish to do so before you try it on the whole lot,—but when testing it, use it as outlined, and do not let the neighbors "butt in."

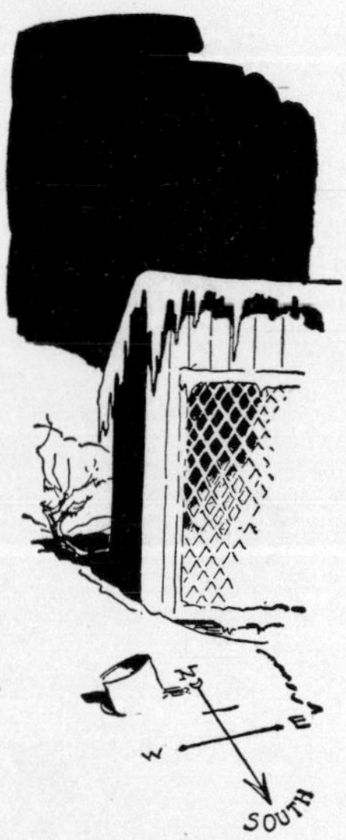

Whether you believe it or not, this is allright.

Results are sure when used as directed, but when diluted and twisted the very purpose for which the strongest features were introduced may be frustrated.

Do not attempt to test out a heatless brooder and put two chickens in it. Neither should you put in twenty-five chickens and then keep them behind a stove. Put twenty-five chickens in the brooder in an unheated room and then follow directions.

Do not take your windows out of your house and then put them in again whenever it looks as though it was going to be a little bit cool, thereby forgetting the principles that fresh air is necessary all the time.

Do not buy Egg Feed and feed it wet, or use inferior brands and mixtures of scratch feeds, thereby throwing the ration out of balance, scouring your birds, and otherwise putting them out of condition.

Do not feed Growing Feed and hope to hasten the growth of your chickens by adding meat food. It should contain all the meat ration necessary for the best results.

Do not have any windows in your breeding pen. Cheese cloth sheeting is much cheaper and means dry, healthy quarters with live air around the stock at all times.

Do not think that you can neglect your stock while it is growing, and get big, robust breeding stock by full feeding a month or so before laying.

Do not expect that you can milk your breeding stock with 50% daily egg yield from December to March, and then get good hatches of chickens that will live.

Do not put ten, twelve, fifteen or twenty females with a male and expect good hatches.

Never put two ages of chickens together in any weather.

Don't put two chickens together where you know you should put one, and don't hesitate to separate them now, not next week.

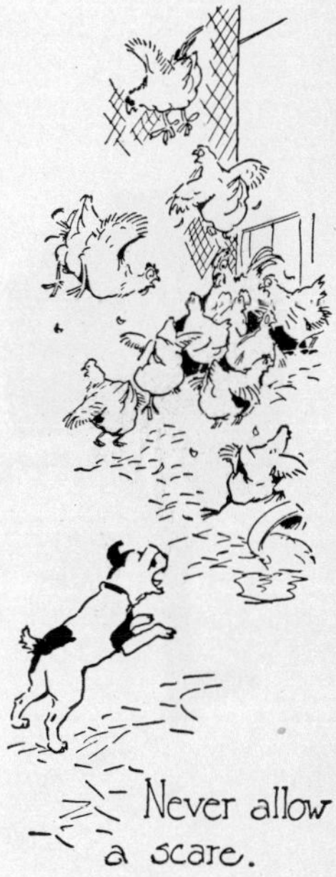